Natural remedies for Lovebirds
Herbal Teas

Copyright © 2017 Erika Busecan

ISBN-13:978-1548426224

ISBN-10:1548426229

Contents

Introduction

In this world, each plant and herb has its own nutritional value and therefore we can use them to heal numerous diseases. All we have to do is to study them and to find out where and when to collect these plants.

If you don't have time to harvest them by your own, then you can buy them from specialized herbal stores. You should always follow the correct dosage that comes along with the indications.

I am using teas especially infusions to prevent and cure possible diseases that may develop in my body and in my bird`s body.

My Lovebirds enjoy drinking these teas and the most important thing is that they look very healthy and happy birds.

A healthy cage bird must have at least 1-3 hours of free flight, for at least three times per week, in order to develop healthy muscles and therefore a healthy organism. The eyes, beak, nostrils, plumage are those factors that indicates if a bird is perfectly healthy.

In this book I will describe several teas that are good for you and also can be offered to your birds as well.

The main purpose of offering tea (infusion) to your bird, is to maintain your bird`s health, well-being and to prevent and cure any kind of diseases.

When our birds are sick, the first thing we are usually doing is we actually visit the vet and ask for help.

In many cases, you will have no choice, but administering antibiotics to your bird.

Taking in consideration that your bird is very sick, only the antibiotics will work against infections caused by bacteria and it is too late to administer herbal teas in the actual state of the bird.

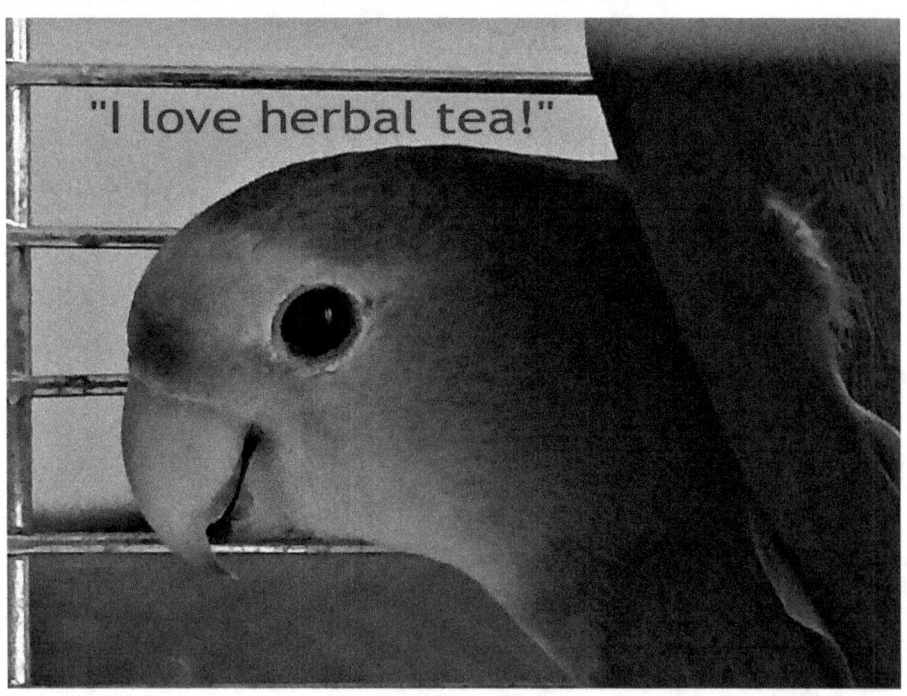

"I love herbal tea!"

You must offer your bird these natural remedies and herbal teas while your bird is perfectly healthy, because this way you can prevent the development of all kind of diseases. Birds usually get sick because their weakened immune system can't fight against the already installed bacteria in their organism.

Consuming herbs and plants does not means that your bird will never get sick, but the purpose of natural remedies and teas intake is to strengthen the bird's immune system, which lead to a healthier life with less medicine and antibiotic in it.

When it comes to our birds health we all know that preventing is always better than curing.

This book comes in the help of Lovebirds lovers that are looking to maintain their bird`s health with 100% natural products, teas.

This presentation will help the birds owners understand how important and how easy is to use these natural products, but most of all how beneficial they are for their beloved birds.

Some of these benefits are: increasing lifespan, immune system enhancement, improved feather growth, color and condition, increasing fertility, healthier offsprings with less deformities and increased survival rate, protection against mycotoxins, prevention of viral and bacterial infections, prevention and treatment of parasites and more.

During egg laying periods the Cuttle fish bone, dried and crushed eggshell, (in this period they need more calcium intake) and most teas like the raspberry tea (is a very good muscle relief) is necessary in the female`s diet. If we don't care for them in egg laying period they will get sick and without proper medical care they could die.

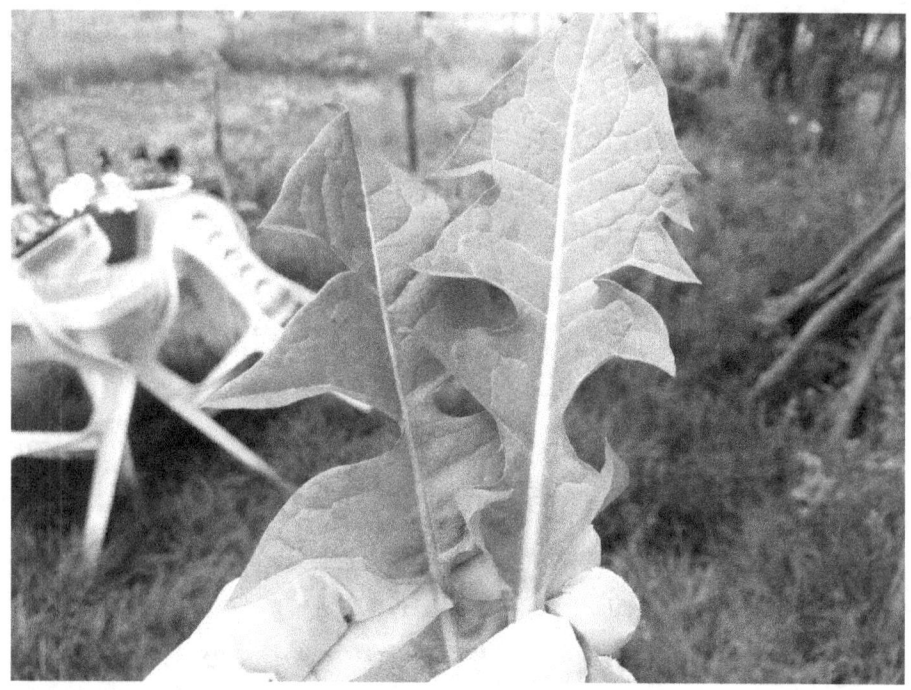

The lack of green leafy vegetables in our birds diet is another detrimental factor which will affect our bird`s health.

Greens are very nutritious and contain almost all the necessary compounds that your bird needs. These greens are: spinach, kale, parsley, beet greens, lettuce, watercress, shepherd`s purse, clover, etc... You can also offer fresh herbs like: dandelion, yarrow (Achillea millefolium), plantain (Plantago lanceolata), coltsfoot (Tussilago farfara), Shepherd's purse (Capsella bursa pastoris), clover. Leaves and branches of fruit trees, oak trees, beech trees (Fagus sylvatica), willow trees (Salix alba) are the best source of vitamins, you can provide them directly from forests. You also have to offer the opportunity to your parrot to chew these kind of branches.

Next, I will present the preparation method of teas (infusion), made from herbs and plants and also 17 types of herbs or plants used for teas, which will make your bird feel much healthier and happier.

How to prepare the infusion

Infusions are typically made with dried or fresh, delicate herbs, plants and leaves. Preparing an infusion is much like making a cup of tea. For fresh herbs, the water is brought just to a boil and then poured over the herb or combination of herbs. It is covered and allowed to steep for 30 seconds - 1 minute or so. It can be prepared in the drinking cup (by just pouring the heated water over the herb in the cup) or by dropping the herb into the pot which the water was heated in. The color of the tea has to be very light, like light yellow or light green. If you prepare the infusion in the heating pan, then it's best to use a ceramic pot with a lid. Stirring it a few times while steeping is helpful. The entire day's dosage can be prepared in the morning (2-3 cups at one time), and the remainder refrigerated until ready to use. The exceptions are the more aromatic plants with active essential oils. These are best prepared in single doses. When you're using dried herbs, leave them to steep for 1 -2 minutes.

You can serve the tea to your bird as soon it has cooled down.

Avoid adding sugar in teas, it is very toxic for your bird!

Kelp or Seaweed

Kelps are seaweeds or brown algae which grow in underwater forests in shallow oceans. Kelp has elongated stem with flat, blade shape leaves.

When consuming kelp, it is very important to know its origin, because as we know many of the world's oceans are polluted. Try to use Kelp products that originates from clean, unpolluted oceans.

Kelp contains carbohydrates, proteins, fats, vitamins as B1 (thiamine), B2 (riboflavin), B3 (niacin), B5 (pantothenic acid), B9 (folate), C, E, K and minerals as zinc, iron, potassium, calcium, phosphorus, magnesium, manganese, sodium. Kelp is very rich in iodine that boost the thyroid gland.

Excessive use of kelp may provide the body with too much iodine and may interfere with thyroid function!

Kelp treat thyroid disorders, rheumatism, constipation, arthritis, obesity, goiter, glandular disorder, poor digestion, high blood pressure, colds, nervous disorders, immune system booster.

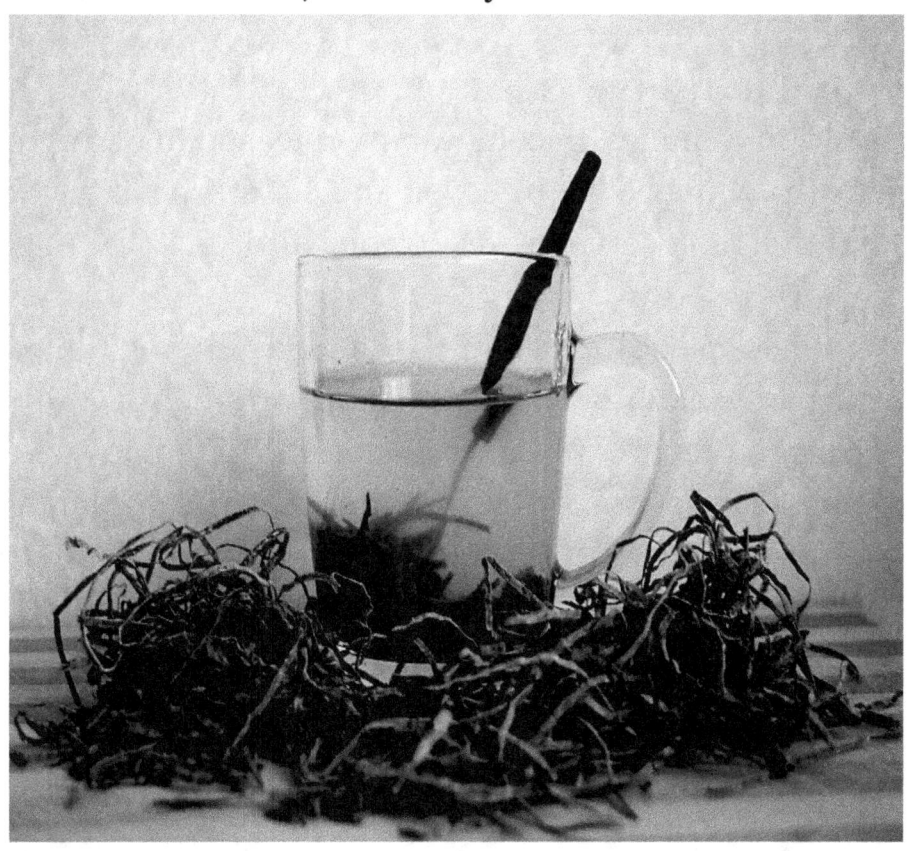

This plant helps prevent the absorption of harmful toxins and chemicals, it reduces the cholesterol level and it has diuretic effect that helps with an irritated bladder.

Kelp maintains the bird's nails, beak and skin in good condition and supports the growth of healthy plumage.

If your bird is suffering from obesity, iodine deficiency, feather plucking, skin problems, colds, rheumatism, constipation, nervous disorder, then you may offer the following cold infusion:

Cold infusion
Add in a mug with cold water 1-2 teaspoon of dried or fresh, chopped kelp, cover and let steep for 1 hour, strain it and serve the tea to your bird.

Kelp powder
The Kelp powder can be added in your bird`s drinking water or it can be mixed with their food.

How to prepare the cold infusion with Kelp powder

Add 1 teaspoon of Kelp powder in a mug, pour cold water, stir it well, let steep for 1 hour and serve it to your bird.

How to prepare the kelp powder with the food

Fill a 250 ml cup with Lovebirds seed mix, drip 5 drops of olive or grape seeds oil on the seeds, mix well with a spoon. Add ½ (half) teaspoon of Kelp powder, mix the seeds again and serve the seeds to your bird. The remainder should be kept in the fridge, because of the oily texture of the seeds, this mixture may become rancid.

Basil (Ocimum basilicum)

Basil or Ocimum basilicum is a culinary herb, also called the "royal herb" of the mint family Lamiaceae. It is native to India, but today can be found all over the world.

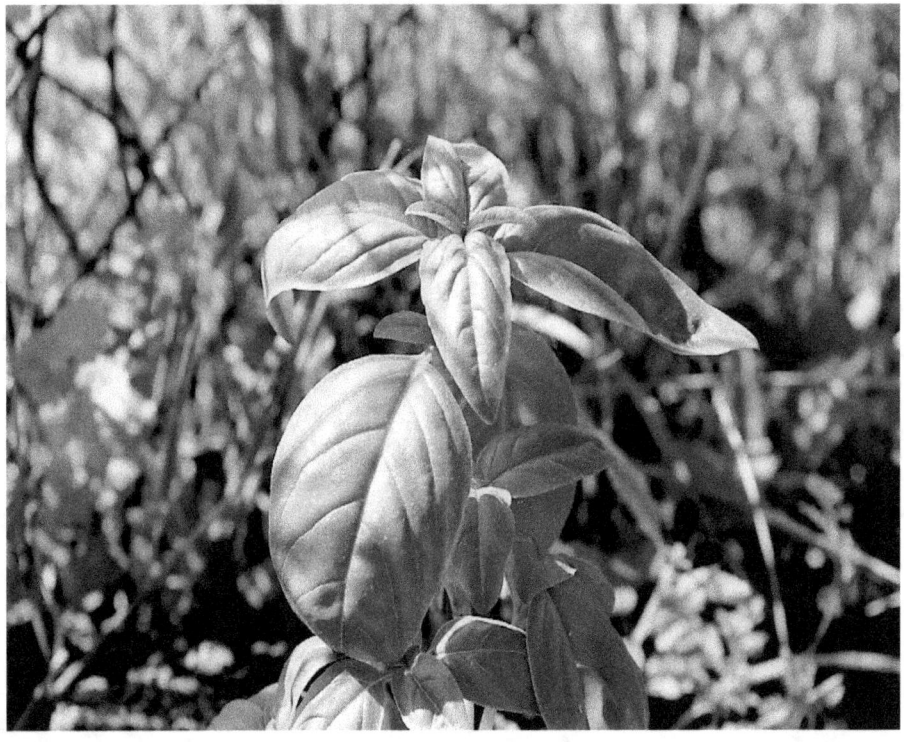

There are several varieties of basil: the sweet basil or Ocimum basilicum (is frequently used in italian cuisine), holy basil (Ocimum tenuiflorum), Thai basil (Ocimum basilicum thyrsiflora), lemon basil (Ocimum citriodorum), etc... The African blue basil (Ocimum Kilimandscharicum) is a perennial plant, while the most common types of basil are considered annual plants.

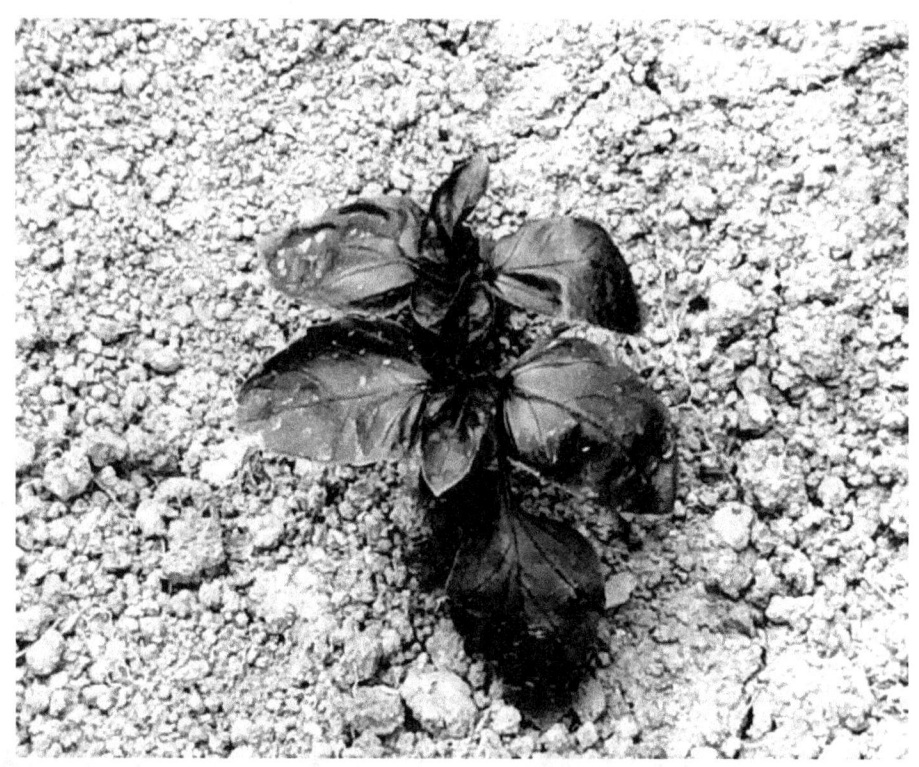

Ocimum basilicum var. purpurascens or "Red Rubin" basil is native to tropical and subtropical Asia.

Basil is a good source of vitamin A, vitamin C, vitamin K, iron, magnesium, calcium and potassium, manganese.

Sweet basil has antibacterial, anti-inflammatory, properties. Sweet basil contains essential oils with phenolic compounds and DNA protecting flavonoids.

Basil treats digestive problems, respiratory diseases, loss of appetite, worm infections, fluid retention, kidney problems, atherosclerosis, lower stress level in loud environments.

How to prepare the sweet basil tea

Add 4-5 fresh, chopped basil leaves in a cup, pour boiling water and steep for 1-2 minutes.

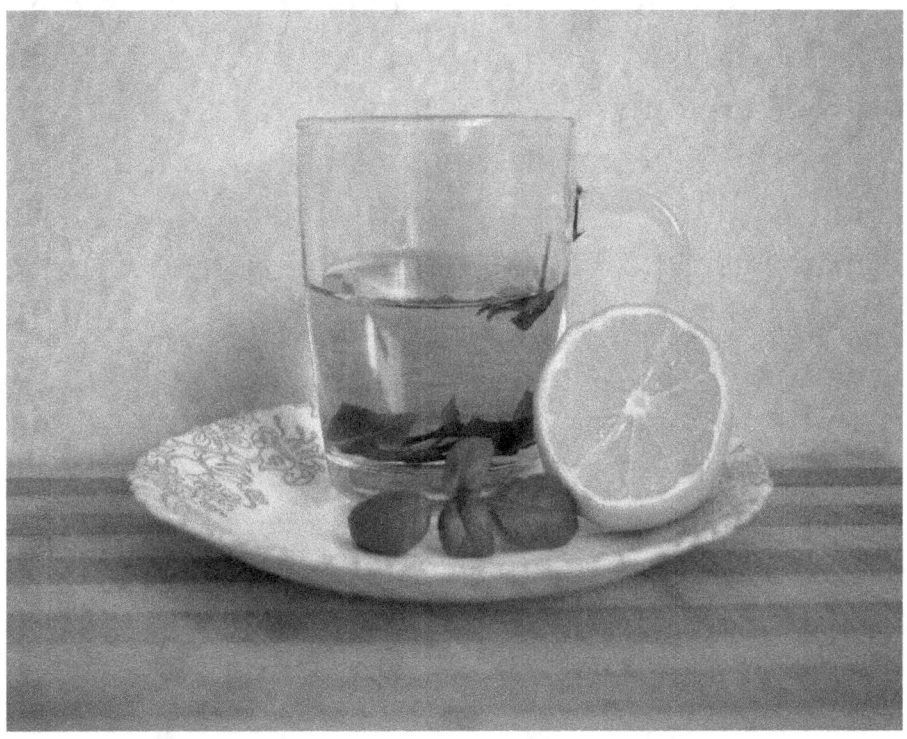

When preparing tea with dried basil leaves, use 1 teaspoon of basil in a cup, steep for 2 minutes, strain it and the tea is ready to serve.

You can use the basil tea if your bird is anxious, stressed or nervous during a trip.

You can also serve it to your bird when she/he is infested with parasites or suffering from respiratory diseases.

Dill (Anethum graveolens)

Dill or Anethum graveolens is an annual herb in the family Apiaceae. It can be found in Europe and Asia. Dill can grow up to 50 cm (20 in), it has finely divided, softly delicate green leaves and yellow flowers. Dill contains vitamins like A, B1, B2, B3, B5, B6, B9, B12, vitamin C, and minerals like calcium, manganese, zinc, phosphorus, potassium, iron, magnesium, and sodium. Dill has carminative, antimicrobial, digestive, disinfectant, antifungal, anti-inflammatory, anti congestive, antihistaminic, antispasmodic, antioxidant, cancer protection, relaxant properties. It is also a very good immune system booster.

Dill increases urination and therefore helps to eliminate the toxins, water and excess salts from the body.

Dill has a good source of calcium and ensures the bones and teeth health.

It is a very good remedy against osteoporosis and is protecting you and your bird from the loss of bone minerals density and it also has the ability to heal injured bones.

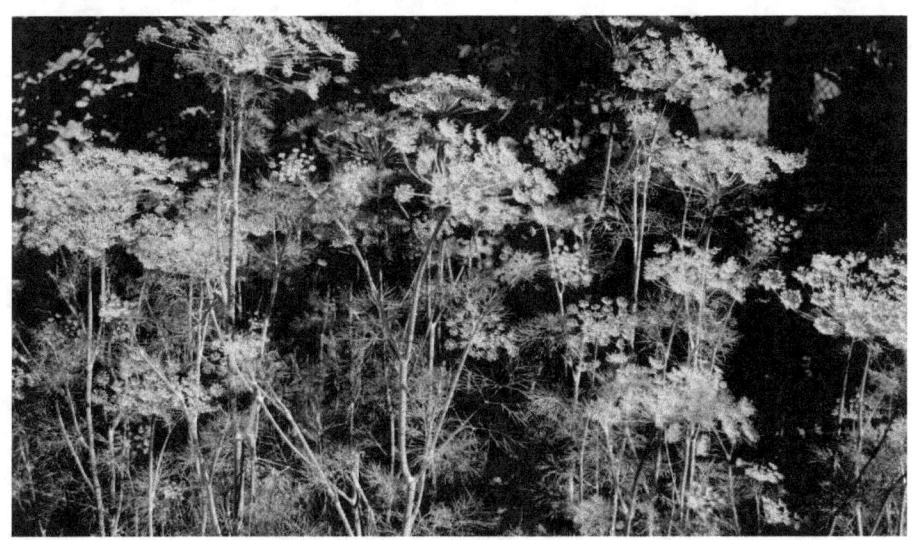

If your bird has injured bones, after a veterinary consultation and care, 2-3 cups of dill tea daily, would be well-coming.

Dill tea is good to treat diarrhoea by stopping the formation of microbial infections which may occur in the body.

The leaves and the seeds are very good mouth and breath fresheners especially in humans.

Those birds which are kept in indoor aviaries or cages usually suffer from calcium deficiency, therefore it is recommended to use this herb as often as possible in their diet.

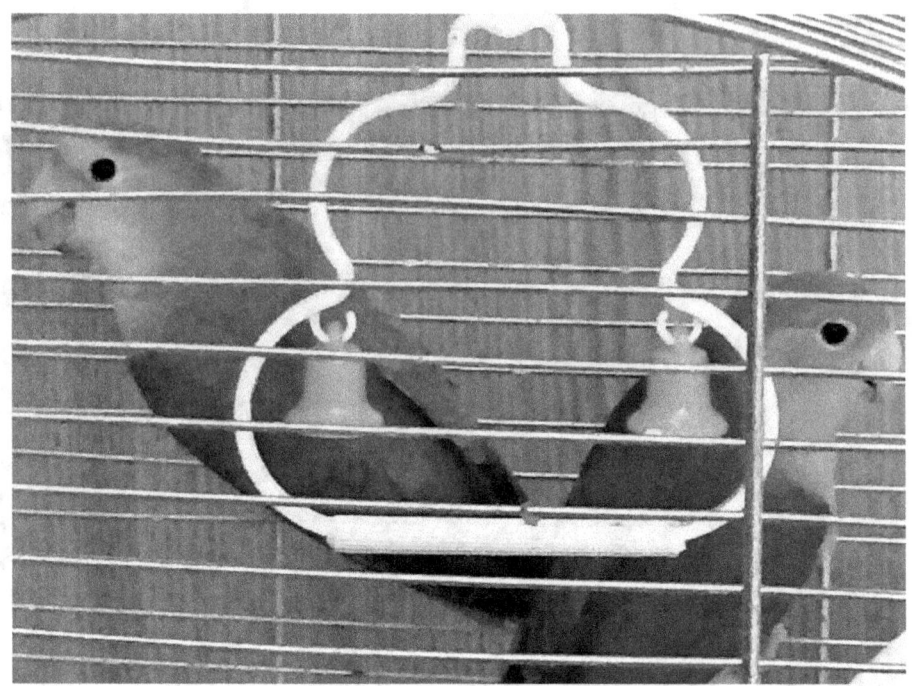

If you grow this excellent herb in your garden it would be good to cut some dill flowers, stems and leaves and give them to your bird. Just tear the flowers in small pieces, chop the leaves and stems and place them in the bird's feeding bowl. Maybe they won't like it for the first time, but after a while they will get used with the taste of this aromatic herb. The chopped dill can be added in their vegetable mixture, as well.

How to prepare the dill tea

Add 2 teaspoon of fresh, chopped dill in a cup, pour boiling water and let steep for 30 seconds - 1 minute.

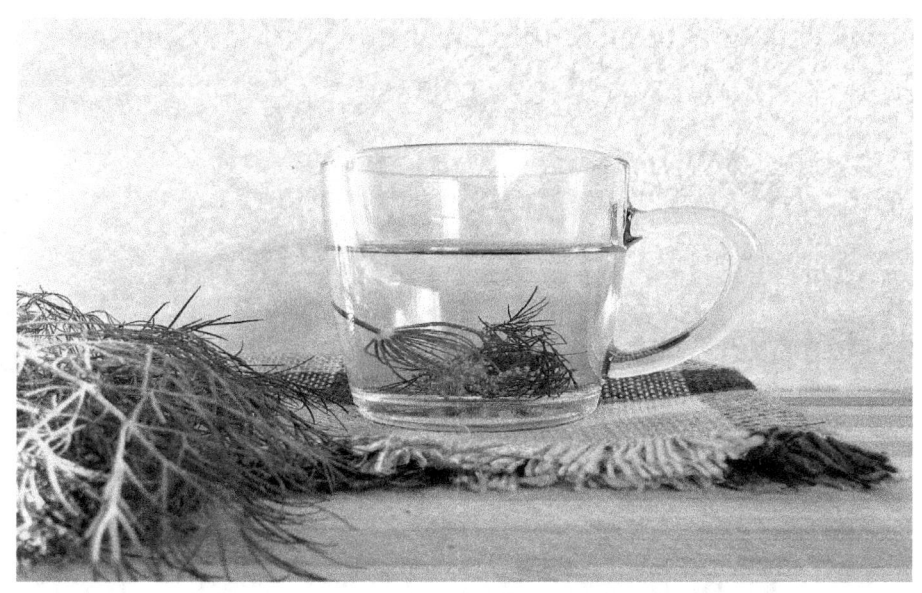

When preparing the tea with dried herbs, add 1 teaspoon of dill in a cup, pour boiling water and let steep for 1-2 minutes.

After it cools down it can be added in the bird's drinking bowl. You can offer your bird this pleasant tasting tea 2-3 times per day for 3-4 days per week.

Oregano (Origanum vulgare)

Oregano or Origanum vulgare is a perennial, flowering herb in the mint family Lamiaceae.

This aromatic herb is native to the Mediterranean and the western and southwestern Eurasia. Oregano has purple flowers and opposite, green leaves and it can grow from 20-80 (7.9-31.5 in) cm tall. Oregano is relative to the herb marjoram or wild marjoram.

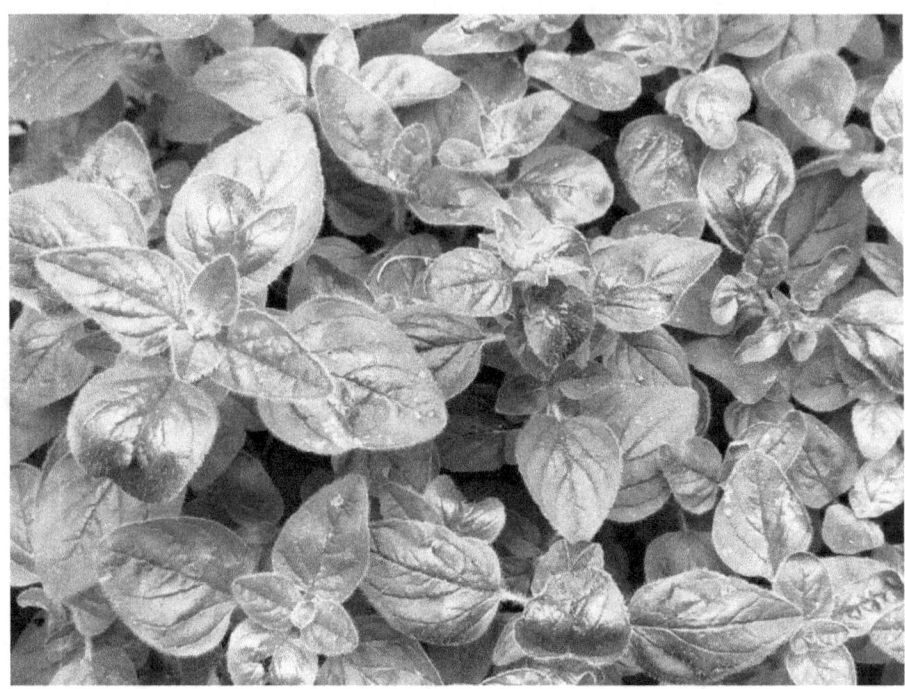

Oregano has antioxidant, antiseptic, anti-cancer, diuretic, expectorant, antibacterial properties. The oregano compounds help prevent the growth of potentially harmful microorganisms. It contains vitamins like vitamin A, C, E and minerals like magnesium, copper, potassium, calcium, zinc, iron, manganese and niacin. Oregano treats the common cold, asthma, bronchitis, stimulates appetite, eliminates intestinal parasites, breaks up nasal congestion, etc..

If your bird suffer from one the symptoms presented above, then you should administer the oregano tea

2-3 times per day for about 1 week to your bird.

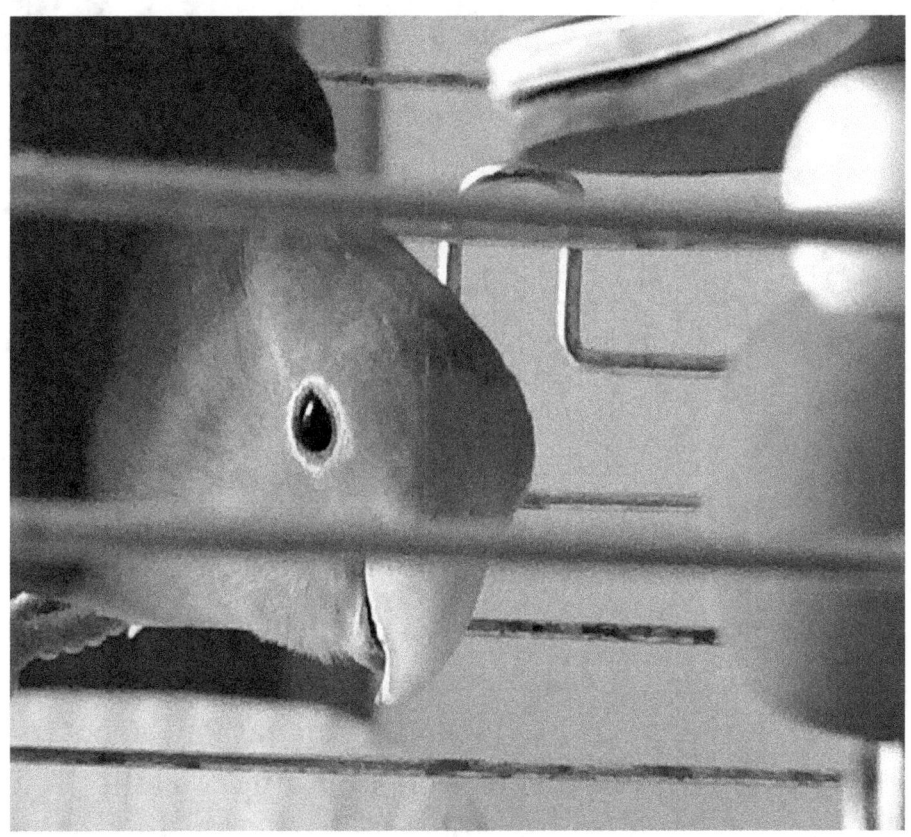

How to prepare the oregano tea

Steep about 10 fresh leaves of oregano in 1 cup of boiling water for 30 seconds or 1 minute.

When making tea with dried oregano leaves, steep 5 dried leaves or 1 teaspoon of oregano in 1 cup of boiling water for 1-2 minutes.

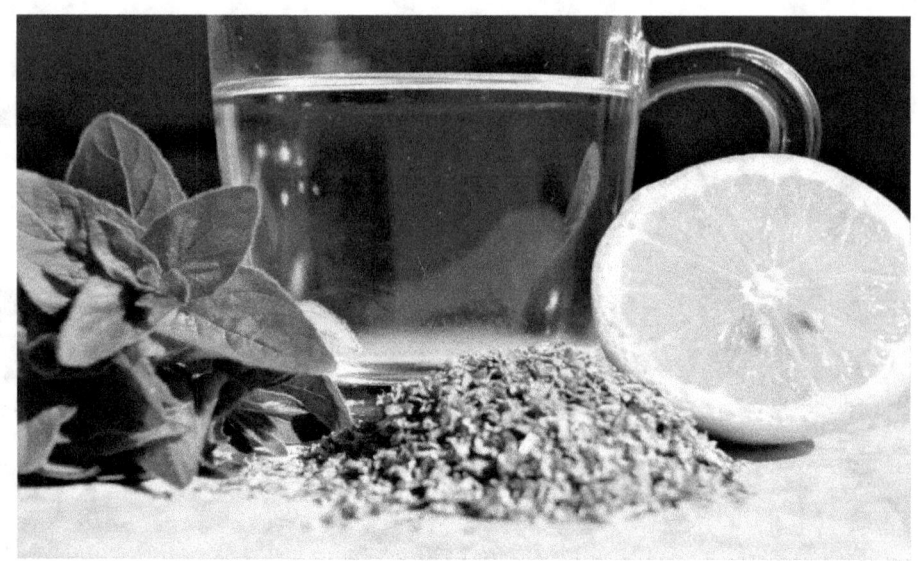

Some birds have a very big appetite, but they'll remain still skinny, because they probably suffer from parasitic infestation (with Dermanyssus gallinae). You can also check your bird`s droppings to see if there are any visible parasites or parasite eggs in it. Even if you don't detect anything in the bird's droppings, you should follow a 1 week treatment with oregano tea.

If your bird is still sick or still eliminates parasites, then you should continue the treatment with green garlic tea for another week.

Green garlic (Allium sativum)

Garlic or Allium sativum is native to central Asia and belongs to family Amaryllidaceae. Green garlic is an immature or young garlic plant that is harvested before it begins to form mature cloves or bulbs. Green garlic is also known as Spring garlic and it is available from late Spring through early Summer.

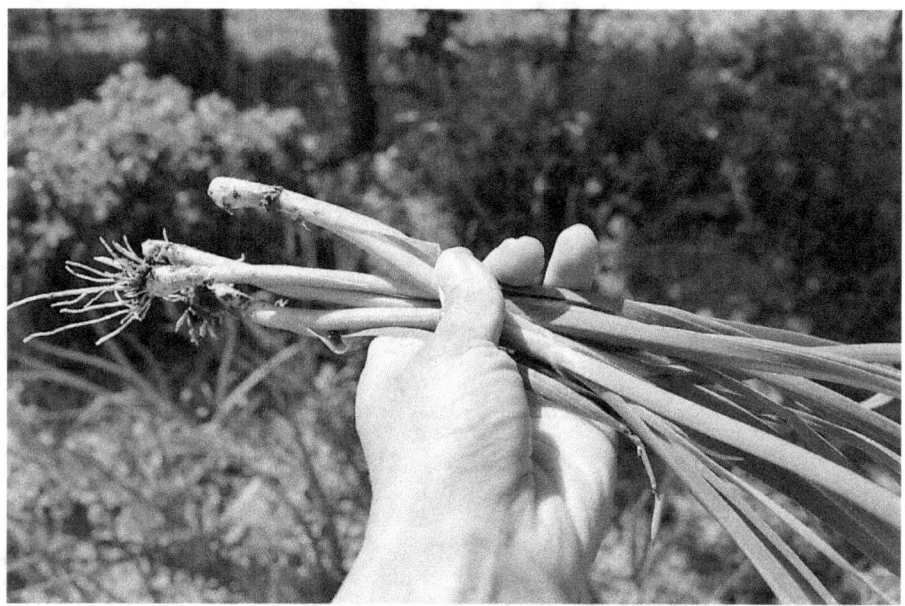

Green garlic is entirely edible, the immature bulb and the green leaves can be used as food flavoring and as a traditional medicine. Green garlic has antibiotic, decongestant, anti-inflammatory, and expectorant properties. It is also used as a diuretic agent, lowers blood pressure and cholesterol, treats the common cold, cancer and eliminates intestinal parasites. Garlic contains vitamin C and B1 (thiamine), B2 (riboflavin), B3(niacin), B5 (pantothenic acid), B6, B9 (folate) and minerals like iron, calcium, manganese, phosphorus and zinc.

It is a perfect immune system booster that has been used for centuries to treat all kind of diseases in birds.

How to prepare the green garlic tea

Place the fresh, young leaves and the bulb of a green garlic in a mug, pour boiling water and cover the mug for 1 minute. Quickly cool it down and add the garlic tea in the drinking bowls.

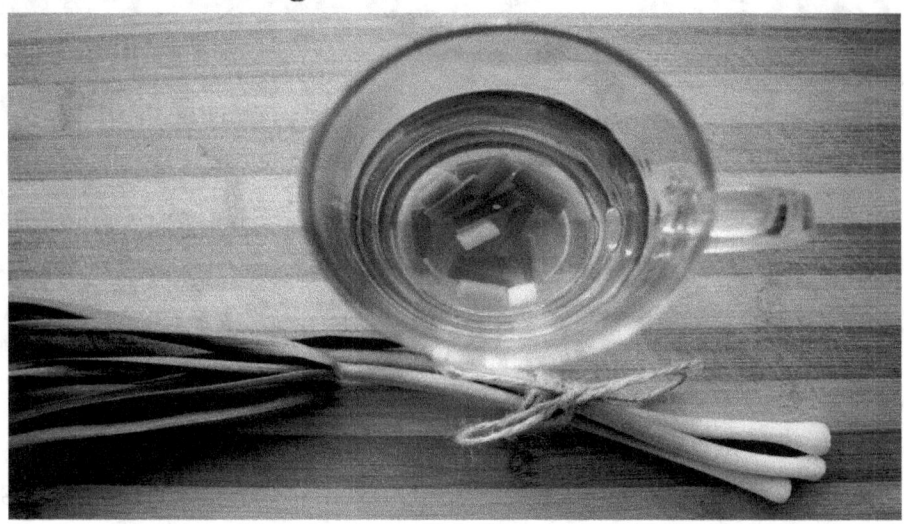

You can give this tea 3 times per day for about a week to your bird. At the beginning the birds might refuse to drink it, but after a few days they will enjoy it and in the end they will love it.

If you don't have green garlic, then you can use normal garlic.

You can also give your bird 1 thin slice of garlic once per week.

Mint (Mentha)

Mint is an aromatic perennial herb which belong to the Lamiaceae family. There are several species: peppermint, spearmint, chocolate mint, wild mint, garden mint, gray mint, Asian mint, Australian mint, etc...

The mint can be found in many environments, but especially in moist soils. It has a strong aromatic odour and a fresh, minty taste. Some species grow naturally along the banks of streams, on the field or in the garden. The mint leaves usually have dark green color, but its color also can vary from gray-green to purple. This plant can grow 10-100 cm tall and it has white or purple flowers. Mint has beneficial properties and helps with digestion, nausea, depression, respiratory disorders and coughs, diarrhea.

When you are travelling long distances with your birds it is good to have with you a plastic bottle filled with unsweetened mint tea. The essential oil from the mint is very soothing for motion sickness and nausea. Just fill their drinking bowls in their cages or carriers for a few minutes, make sure that they are drinking some tea and then throw away the rest of it.

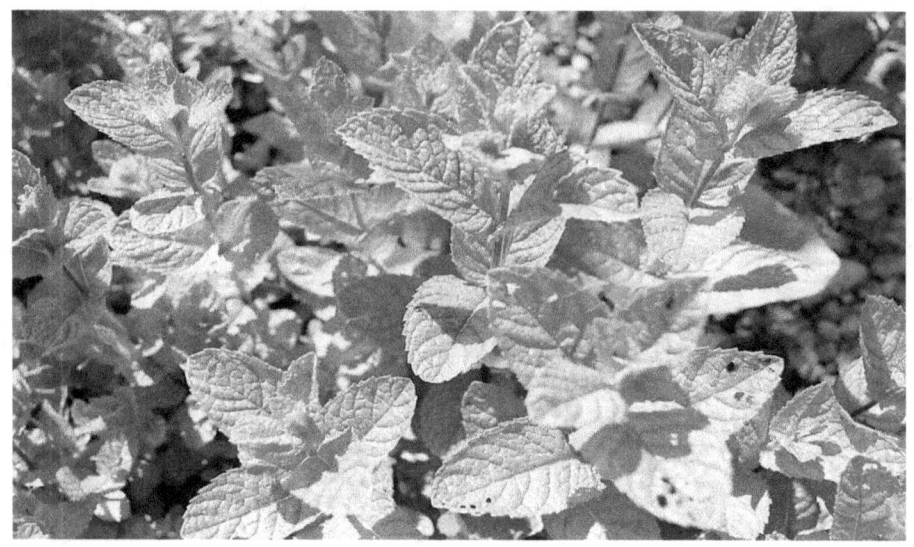

It may be possible that your bird is refusing to drink the mint tea during the trip, in this case, serve your bird only mint tea, one day before the trip, because it will help your bird with nausea and an upset stomach.

Mint tea is also good against diarrhoea, so when you observe that your bird`s droppings are very soft even fluid, with a smell and color different from normal, then you should give your bird instead of water only mint tea 2-3 times per day for 3-4 days or until the bird is healed.

In this period you should feed your bird some poppy seeds, because of their calming effect and mashed boiled rice with some coal powder in it.

When your bird is eating fruits, its droppings become

more watery, but this should not cause alarm. (this situation should not have been confused with diarrhoea).

Mint is a natural stimulant, so if your bird is suffering from depression and it looks exhausted, mint tea can help. Give your bird mint tea once per day for 2-3 days. You can repeat this procedure after 3 days.

Mint tea clears up congestion of nose, throat and lungs so it is a good remedy for respiratory disorders, like common cold and asthma. Offering mint tea 2-3 times per day for 6-7 days should make your bird feel much better.

Asthma is a common disease even among cage birds. It is a lung and respiratory disease which causes an allergic reaction in the bird's body. The symptoms include breathing difficulty, watery eyes, nasal discharge, and sneezing. The common cause of asthma among cage birds is the powder down produced by the feather dust of the birds. Overcrowded, unventilated aviaries may be the sources of such illness as asthma.

Lovebirds may develop this disease, if they live in overcrowded aviaries among other parrot species. Some parrot species like African Grey parrots and Cockatoos are likely to produce this feather dust that can cause allergies, if their environment is not properly cleaned.

The suffering bird has to be isolated in a clean, well ventilated place and the following treatment must be applied: the watery eyes and the nasal discharge must be cleaned with chamomile tea daily by using an eyedropper. Drip 2 drops in each eyes and in each nostril 2-3 times per day for a week. In this period replace the drinking water with mint tea for 2 times per day. After one week try to observe the bird's health progress. If the symptoms still persist then repeat the treatment for another week.

Avoid using cosmetic products (deodorants, hair lacquer, nail polish remover) and any other chemicals (paints, diluents, diesel, gasoline, bleach) in the presence of your bird. These toxic products can cause asthma and even death!

How to prepare the mint tea

Tear 4-5 fresh mint leaves with your hands and place them in a cup. Pour the boiling water over the leaves, cover the tea cup and let the leaves steep for 30 seconds - 1 minute. You can serve the tea to your birds while it is warm or at room temperature (avoid giving hot tea to your bird!).

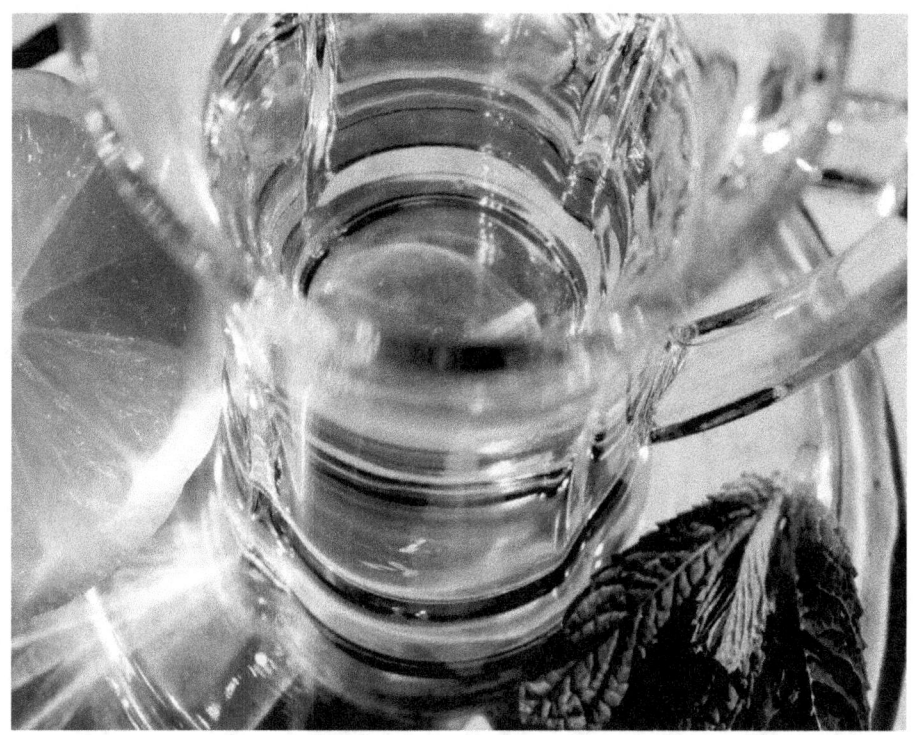

To quickly cool down the hot tea, add cold water in a tea pan (a deep pan used to make tea) and put the cup in the pan and stir it with a teaspoon. After 1-2 minutes just take out the cup from the pan, replace the warm water from the pan with cold water and put the cup back in the pan and leave it for another 1-2 minutes.

Always strain the tea and taste it with a teaspoon to check the temperature of the tea before give it to your bird. You can always stand it in cold water for more or less time to suit you.

Avoid using glass - cups or water glasses when you try to cool down your tea. The overheated glass will crack with the contact of the cold water!

When you prepare the tea with dried mint, add 1 teaspoon of mint in the cup, pour boiling water, cover the teacup and let the dried herbs steep for 1-2 minutes. Strain it, cool it down and pour it into your bird`s drinking bowl.

Stinging Nettle (Urtica dioica)

Nettle or stinging nettle is a herbaceous perennial flowering plant that belongs to the family Urticaceae.

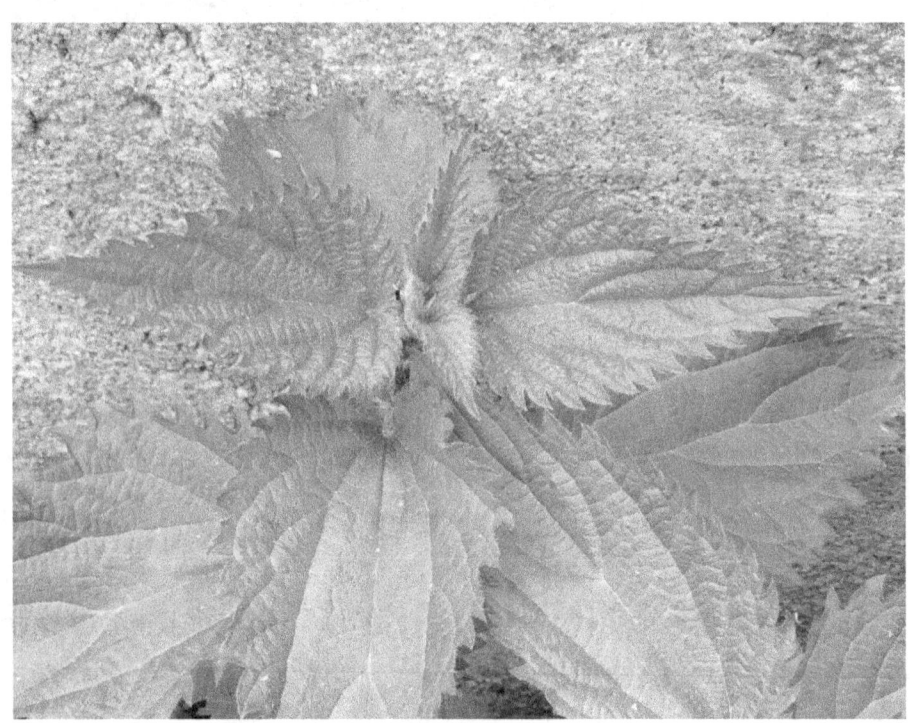

It can be found almost all over the world and it is divided in six subspecies. Urtica dioica or stinging nettle can grow up to 2 meters (7 feet) tall and it has green leaves and stems with stinging hairs.

The stinging hairs contain several substances like histamine, acetylcholine, leukotrienes, moroidin and make the nettle a valuable plant for its curative properties. Stinging nettle has the following medicinal qualities: antiviral, diuretic, antifungal, antibacterial, nutrient, tonic, anti-rheumatic, kidney depurative, blood purifier, hypoglycemic, anti-spasmodic, stimulant, haemostatic, etc...

It contains vitamin A, B complex, C, K and minerals like iron, magnesium, potassium and is a very good Spring tonic for your birds, especially for the females. It is also recommended before, during and after egg laying period.

Nettle is a rich source of iron and should be consumed especially by those birds that are suffering from anaemia or iron deficiency. This herb is also good to treat gout, urinary retention, inflammation of the bladder, kidney stones, hay fever, seasonal allergies, asthma, eczema.

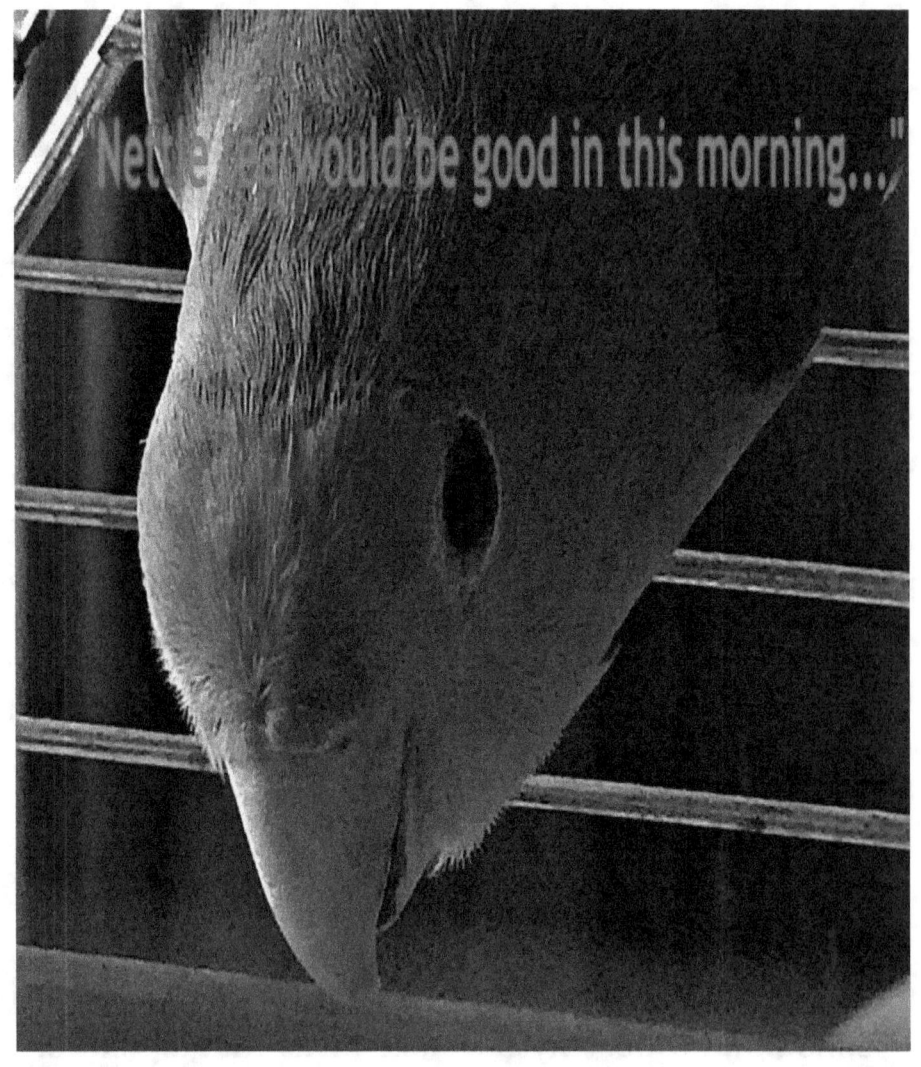

"Nettle tea would be good in this morning..."

How to prepare the stinging nettle tea

Add 4-5 fresh nettle leaf in a cup. Pour the boiling water over the leaves, cover the tea cup and let the leaves steep for 30 seconds - 1 minutes. You can serve the tea to your birds warm or at room temperature.

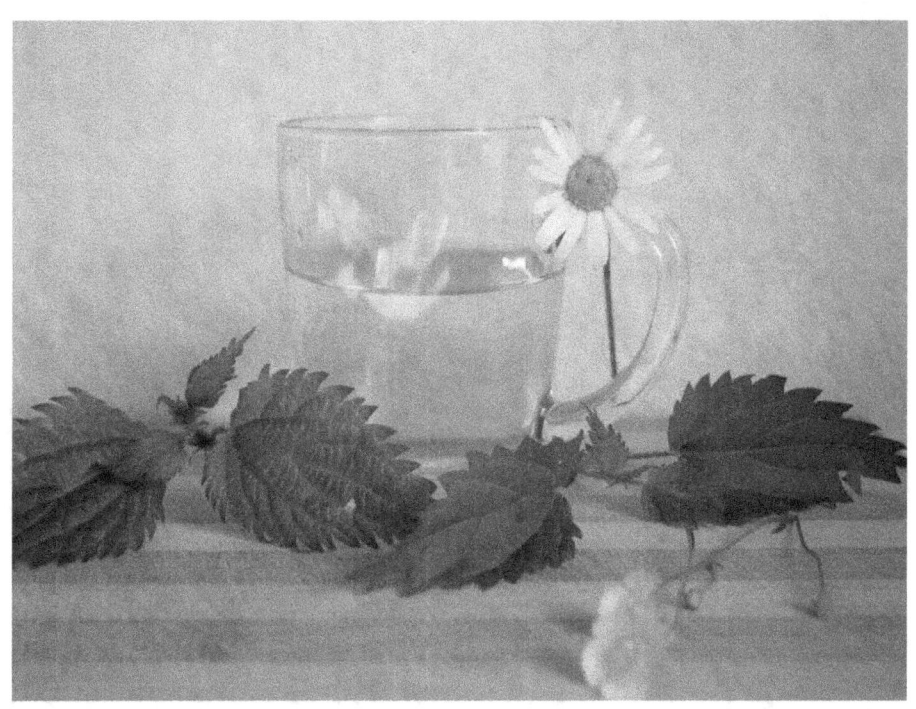

When preparing tea with dried nettle, put 1 teaspoon of nettle in a cup, pour boiling water and let steep for 1-2 minutes. Strain it, cool it down and pour it into your bird`s drinking bowl.

Fennel (Foeniculum vulgaris)

Fennel or Foeniculum vulgaris is a perennial plant with yellow flowers and green feathery leaves.
It is native to the shores of the Mediterranean, but it also can be found almost all over the world. Fennel belongs to the parsley family, called Umbelliferae. It is a very aromatic herb and it is used in culinary and medicinal purposes.

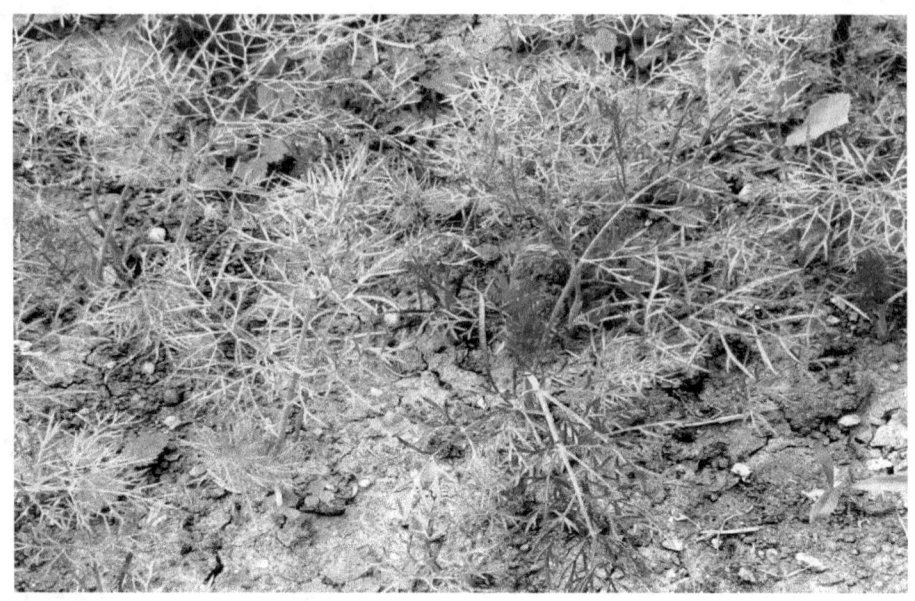

Fennel seeds contain proteins, fibers, carbohydrates, vitamin A, B, C, E and minerals like iron, zinc, copper, selenium, manganese, calcium and magnesium. It also contains volatile oils compounds such as anethole, myrcene, anisic aldehyde, fenchone, chavicol, cineole, etc...

The fennel seeds are almost similar in appearance and taste with anise seeds, therefore these seeds can be confused very easily.

Fennel is used for different health problems like heartburn, gastrointestinal inflammations, digestive disorders, loss of appetite, visual problems, coughs, upper respiratory tract infections, bronchitis, etc...

Fennel is also good as an antidote to cure intoxications with poisonous plants, snake bites and poisonous mushrooms.

How to prepare the fennel tea

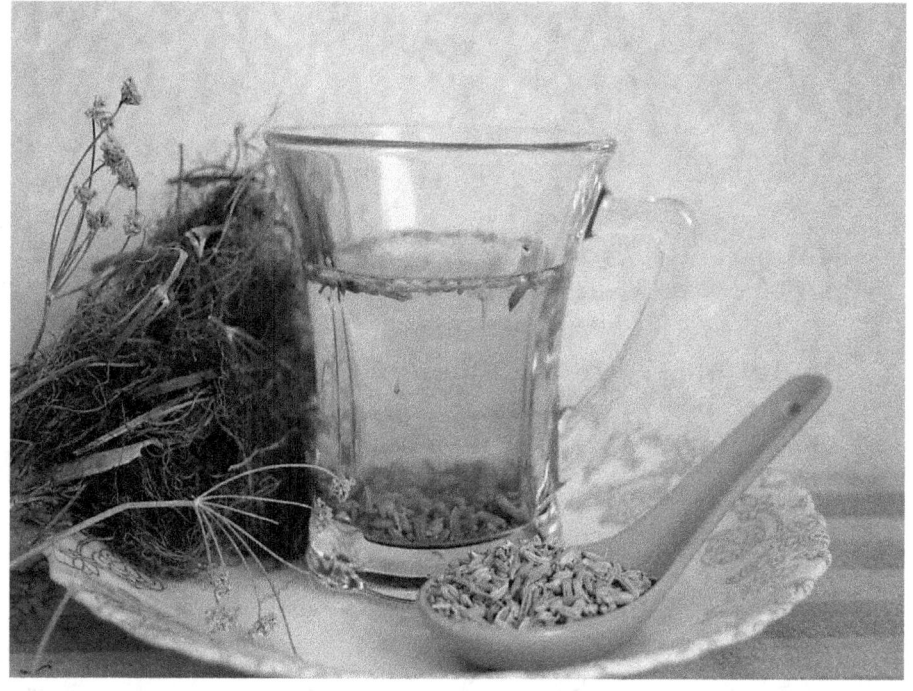

Add 2 teaspoon of fresh leaves, stems and seeds in a mug, pour boiling water and let steep for 1 minute.

When preparing the tea with dried fennel seeds, add 1 teaspoon of fennel seeds in a mug, pour boiling water and let steep for 2 minutes.

This refreshing tea is recommended to be consumed in the mornings.

Chamomile (Matricaria Chamomilla)

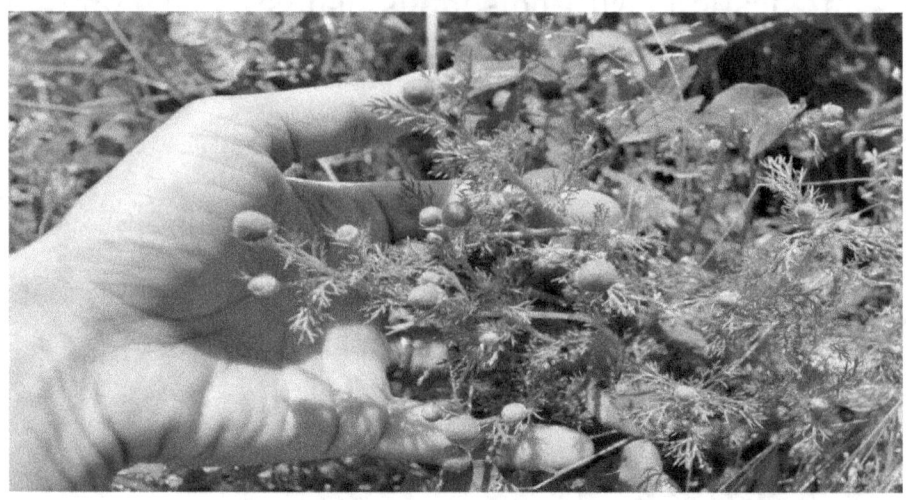

Chamomile is a medicinal herb with daisy-like flowers which is a member of the Asteraceae family.

These daisy-like flowers are very rich in essential oils, matricin, bisabolol, flavonoids and other substances. Chamomile contains substances with powerful anti-inflammatory, antispasmodic, antibacterial, antipyretic, antifungal and anti allergenic effect. There are many different species of Chamomile, but the two commonly used species are: German chamomile (Matricaria Chamomilla) and Roman Chamomile (Chamaemelum nobile).

German chamomile is an annual plant and it has a sweeter taste, than the Roman chamomile which is a perennial plant and it has a bitter taste when used in teas.

German chamomile can be used internally and externally. Chamomile tea can be used with success in insomnia, stomach and intestinal pains, abdominal spasm, inflammation, nervous complaints, fever, asthma, skin diseases, rheumatic problems and rashes, wounds, burns, hemorrhoids, etc...

Chamomile vapors can be used to heal cold symptoms and asthma. Chamomile tea can be used as a compress for skin problems and as a wash for inflammation of mucous tissue.

If your bird has irritated, infected eyes or suffering from conjunctivitis, then you should use a compress with chamomile tea (at room temperature) or you can use an eyedropper. Just fill the dropper with chamomile tea and drip 2-3 drops on the affected eye.

To break up nasal congestion during a common cold, just drip 2 drops of warm (not hot!) chamomile tea in each nostril of the bird.

Abundant nose secretions

The secretion which appears at nose area indicates that the bird is cold sick. You should maintain the bird's body temperature by covering it with a piece of cotton cloth.

There are lots of secretion in the nose when the bird is suffering from mycotic, bacterial and viral infestations.

You have to avoid the contact of your bird with other cage birds and you'll have to feed the bird with soft food, seeds soaked in milk, honey and chamomile tea. In this period vitamins A, C, and B complex intake is needed.

When your bird is suffering from diarrhoea and the vent area is very dirty, wash this area first with warm water, then use a compress and wash it again but this time use warm chamomile tea.

During egg laying period it is good to have chamomile tea instead of water in the drinkers, because the chamomile has the ability to relax the muscles of the uterus and helps ease the discomfort of egg laying.

Constipation

The signs of constipation are the enlarged abdomen of the bird, and the missing fresh droppings on the cage floor. The impossibility of elimination of droppings leads to intoxication. In this situation, the cloacal orifice free opening is needed by administering few drops of castor oil through the bird's beak, for two-three days. The bird will need a warm place and for the next few days the diet will contain honey, green plants, fruits and chamomile tea.

How to prepare the chamomile tea

In a cup place 1 teaspoon of fresh chamomile flowers, pour boiling water and let steep for 30 seconds - 1 minute.

When preparing the tea with dried chamomile, just add half a teaspoon of herbs in the cup and let steep for 1 -2 minutes.

Your bird will enjoy the pleasant taste of this aromatic herb.

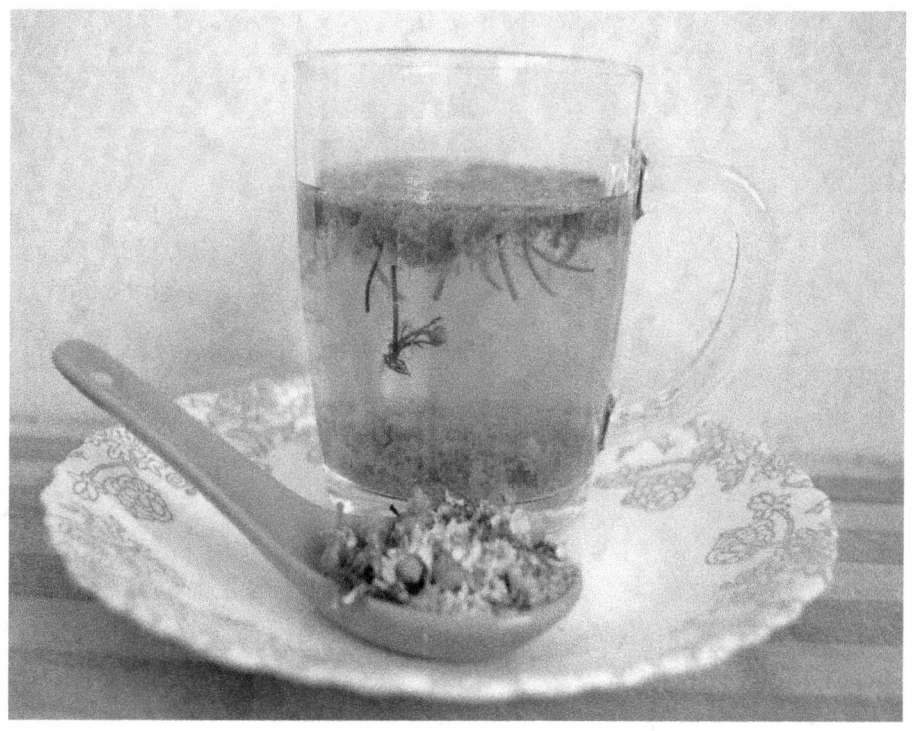

Dandelion (Taraxacum Officinale)

Dandelion (Taraxacum Officinale) are flowering plants in the family Asteraceae. They are native to Eurasia, North and South America, but today they can be found all over the world. All parts of dandelion is edible. It has yellow flowers and green sharp leaves, therefore your bird will love to eat this nutritious plant. Dandelion is used as a tonic and a blood purifier.

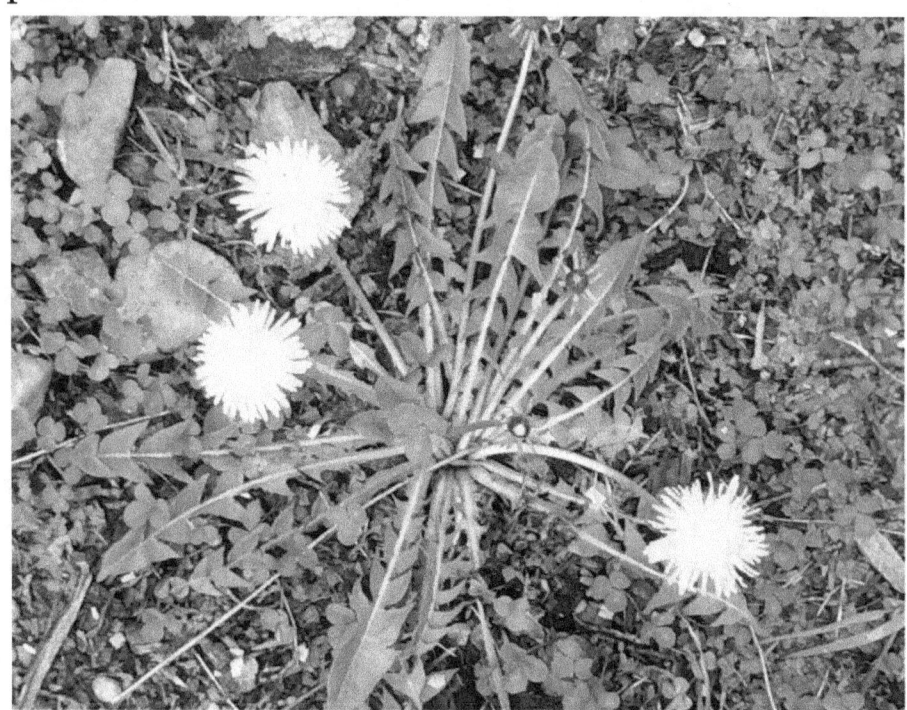

Dandelion leaves contain vitamins A, B, C, K, and minerals like zinc, iron, magnesium, potassium, calcium, choline.

Dandelion is used to cure urinary tract infections, it supports detoxification of the body and healthy liver function, kidney problems, fever, diabetes, urinary infection, gout, eczema and arthritis.

Dandelion is also good to treat obesity. Obesity could lead to health problems like heart and circulatory system disorders, joint problems, modification of the internal organs like fatty liver and constipation.

You should replace the bird's drinking water with dandelion tea, for 20 days. The obese bird will have to receive only half part of the usual daily seeds portion. Green leaves (spinach, lettuce, kale, dandelion, etc...) and fruits can be offered daily.

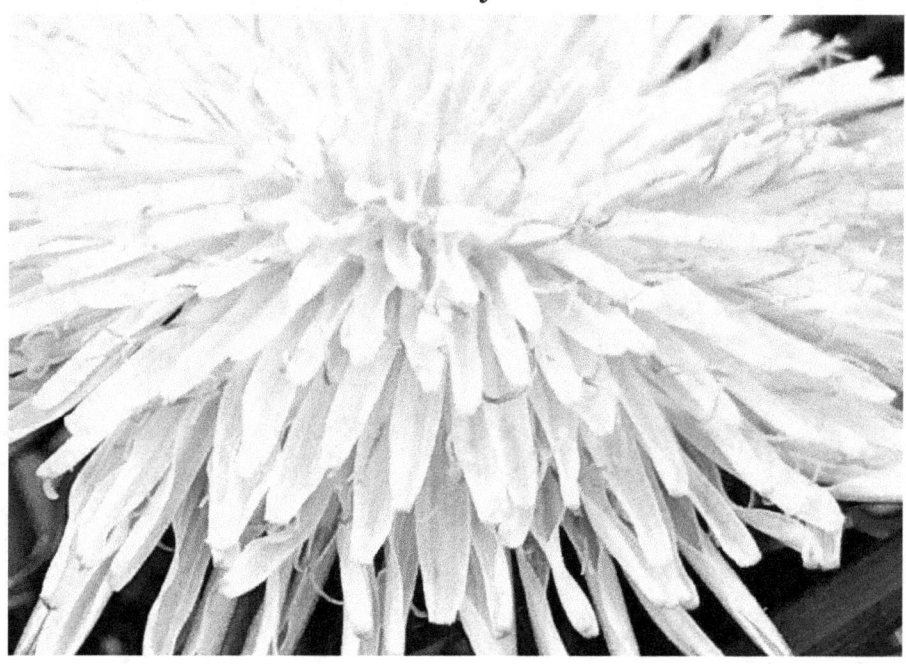

The dandelion tea made from fresh flowers and leaves especially during Spring time is very beneficial for your birds health.

How to prepare the dandelion tea
Add 2-3 fresh, chopped dandelion leaves and flowers in a mug, pour boiling water on them and steep for 2 minutes.

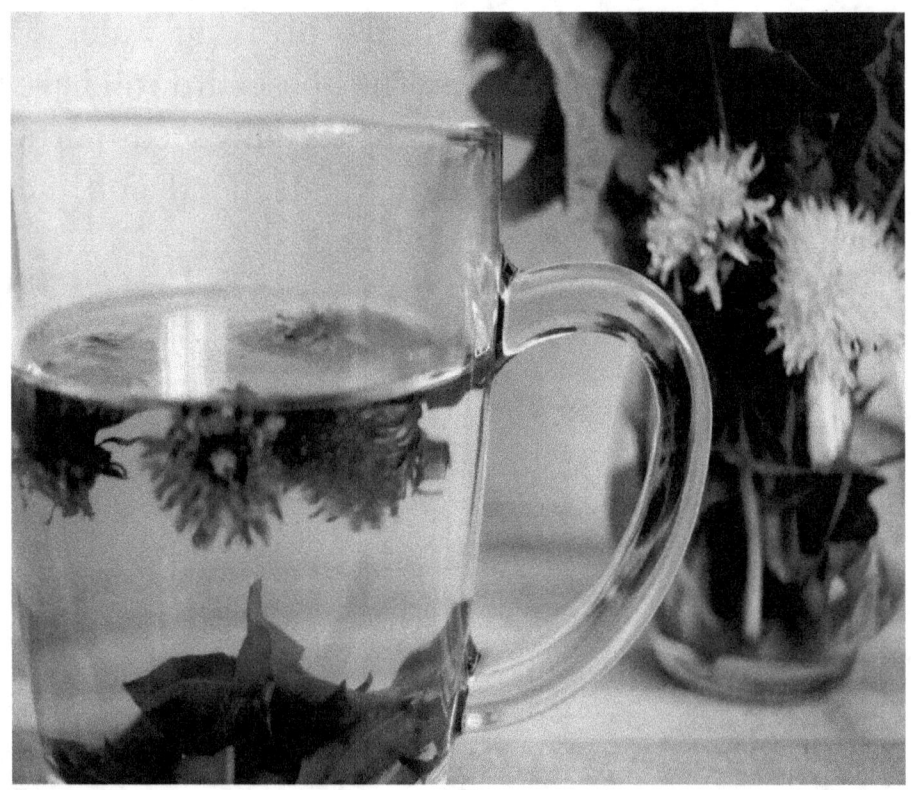

When using dried herbs, add 1 teaspoon of leaves and flowers, pour boiling water and let steep for 3 minutes.

The Norway spruce or Picea Abies

The Norway spruce or Picea Abies is native to Eastern, Central and Northern Europe.

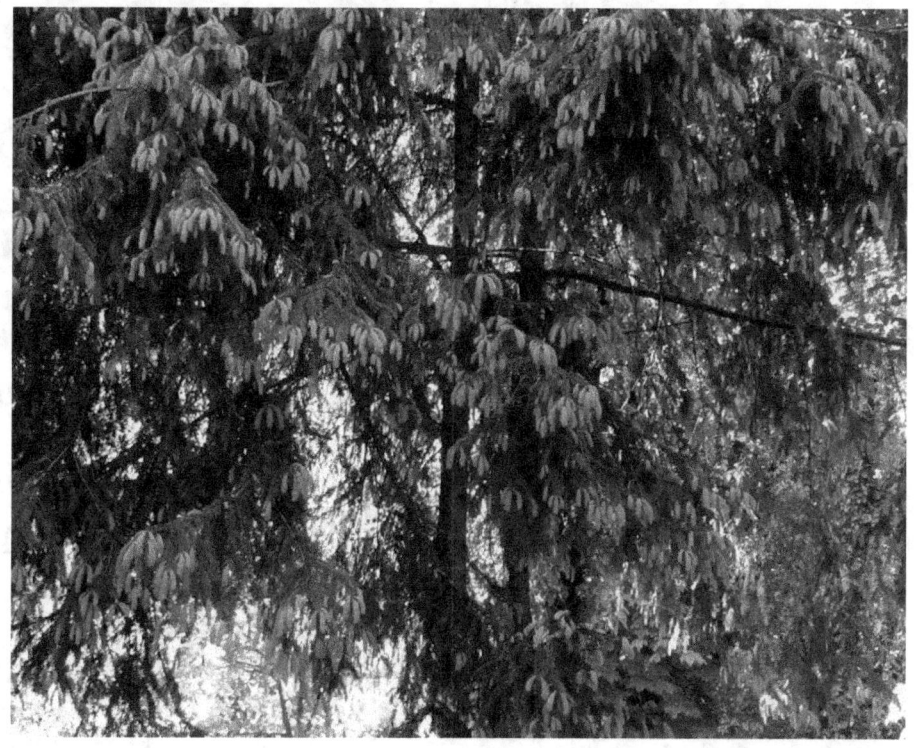

The Norway spruce belongs to the family Pinaceae and is an evergreen coniferous tree that can grow to 115-180 ft (35-55 metres) tall.
The green needle like leaves are flattened and the bark and wood of spruce are rich in antioxidative polyphenols. This tree is commonly used as Christmas tree across Europe.

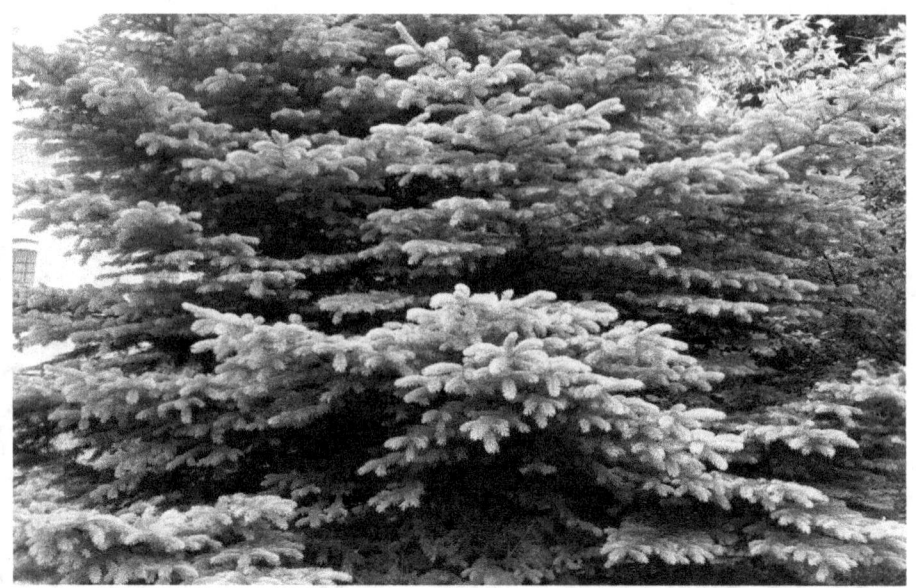

European silver fir, Abies alba. The fresh fir buds from this tree can also be consumed as tea.

A resinous essential oil can be extracted from the needle shaped leaves. In Spring the fresh spruce tips can be consumed as tea or even eaten.

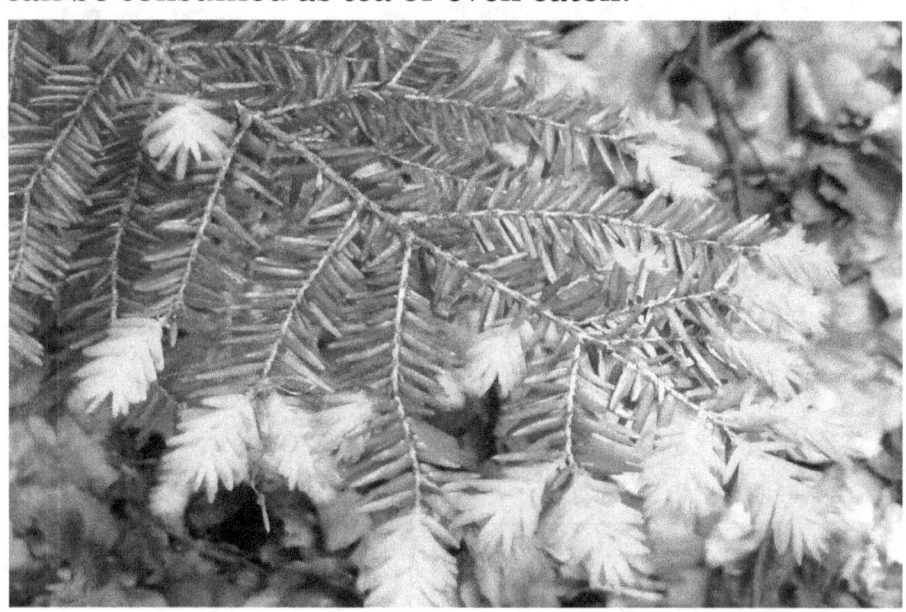

The Norway spruce buds are those young, soft tips of the spruce branches that emerge in Spring. The Norway shoot tips are known to contain very high level of vitamin C and the tea is used for treatment of respiratory tract disorders (the essential oil from the spruce clean and disinfect the lungs), gastrointestinal problems.

It also contains minerals like potassium and magnesium. Because of the high level of chlorophyll, it helps healing tissues and is a very good blood purifier. It also has stimulating, sudorific, antibacterial, mucus dissolvent properties and it treats with success Spring tiredness, asthma, bronchitis, sinus inflammation, gout, rheumatism, neuralgias, etc...

You can use the spruce tips in two ways, by adding them to drinking water or using them for tea.

Cold infusion

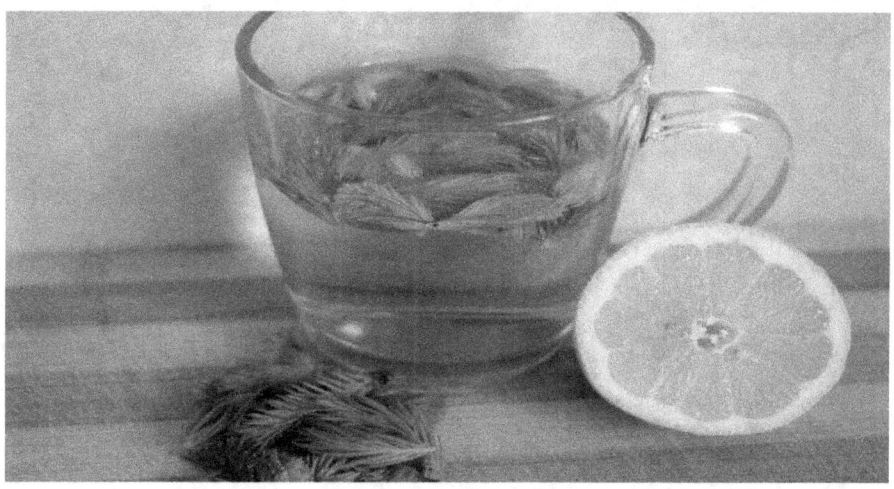

Add 1 tablespoon of fresh, spruce tips in a mug of water, let it sit for 2 hours, strain it and serve it to your birds. The water absorbs all the nutrients from the spruce tips.

How to prepare the Norway spruce tea

Add 1 teaspoon of fresh, spruce tips in a cup, pour boiling water and let steep for 2 minutes.

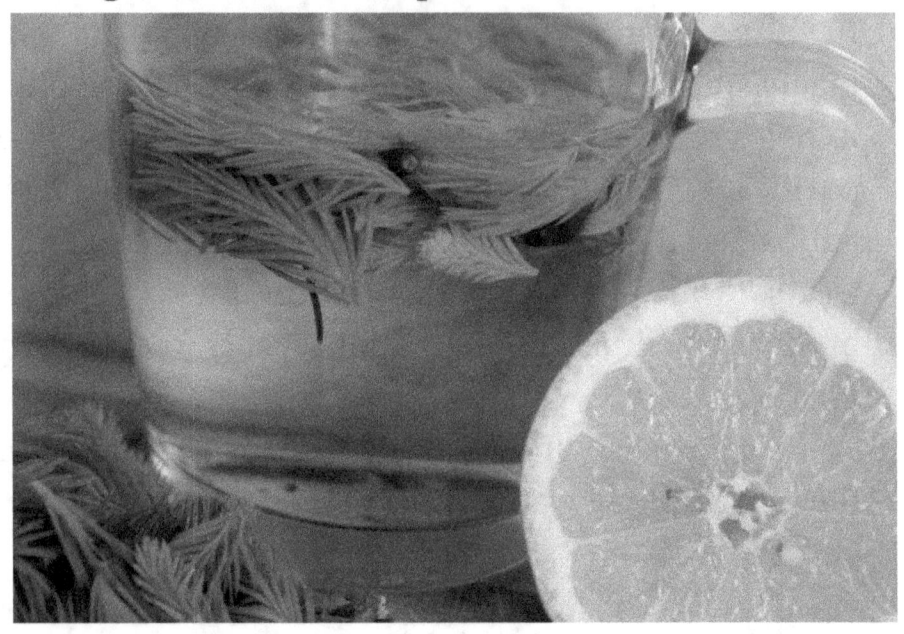

Cinnamon (Cinnamomum verum)

Cinnamon (Cinnamomum verum) is a spice made from the inner bark of several species of trees. The "true" cinnamon is considered to be the best cinnamon and it is called Ceylon cinnamon, while Cassia cinnamon is the more common variety today and it is frequently used for international commerce.

All species of cinnamon trees are members of the genus Cinnamomum in the family Lauraceae.

Cinnamon is native to India, Sri Lanka, Bangladesh and Myanmar.

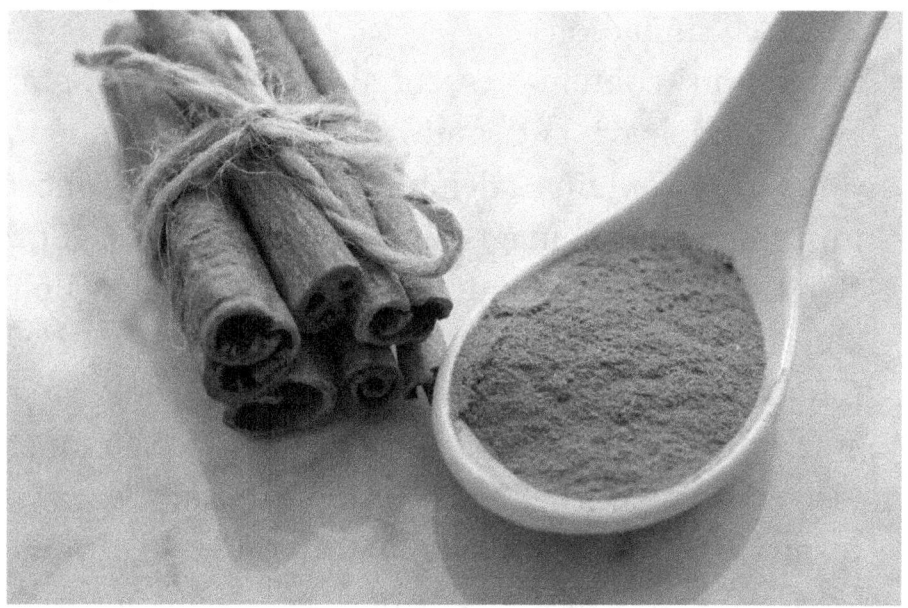

Cinnamon is an evergreen tree with green, oval-shaped leaves, berry fruits and thick bark.

The cinnamon sticks are made by extracting the inner bark from the Cinnamomum tree, the woody parts are removed from it and when it dries, it forms strips that curl into rolls. It is better to use Ceylon cinnamon (the original cinnamon), because the Cassia cinnamon is much higher in coumarin which is believed to be harmful in large doses (it can cause liver damage).

You can check the quality of the cinnamon by doing the following steps:

Just take the end of the stick and crumble a bit into the tea, if it sinks to the bottom, then it is Ceylon cinnamon, the real cinnamon. If your stick isn't the kind that crumbles and is more woody kind, then it isn't real cinnamon.

Cinnamon contains essential oils which contains cinnamaldehyde and antioxidants like polyphenols. Cinnamon contains calcium, potassium, phosphorus, iron, manganese, magnesium and vitamins A, B6, C, E, K, niacin, pantothenic acid, betaine, folate, choline and riboflavin.

Cinnamon has anti-inflammatory, detoxifying, antiviral, antifungal, antibacterial (Salmonella, Listeria) properties. It fights tissue damages, respiratory tract infections, it reduces high blood pressure, heart diseases, it protects against cancer, it protects brain function, is an immune system booster and it has beneficial effect on blood sugar level.

Cinnamon tea has a sweet spice flavor and your birds will love it.

How to prepare the cinnamon tea
Place a cinnamon stick in a mug, pour boiling water and let it steep for 10-15 minutes. Each stick should be good for several uses. I have used one stick three times.

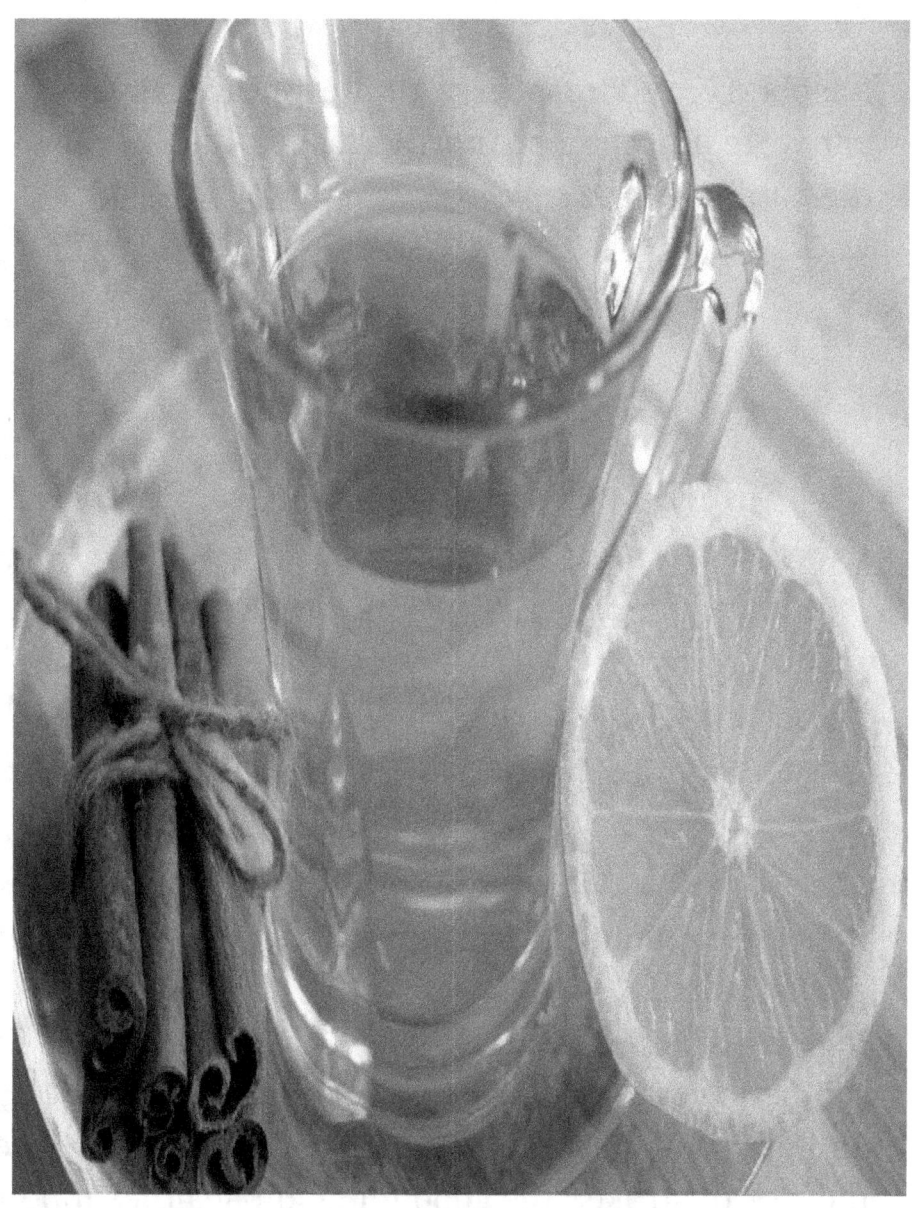

If you are using cinnamon powder, add half a teaspoon of cinnamon powder in a cup, pour boiling water, stir and let steep for 1 minute.

Raspberry (Rubus idaeus)

Raspberry, red raspberry or European raspberry is native to Europe and northern Asia and belongs to the family Rosaceae.

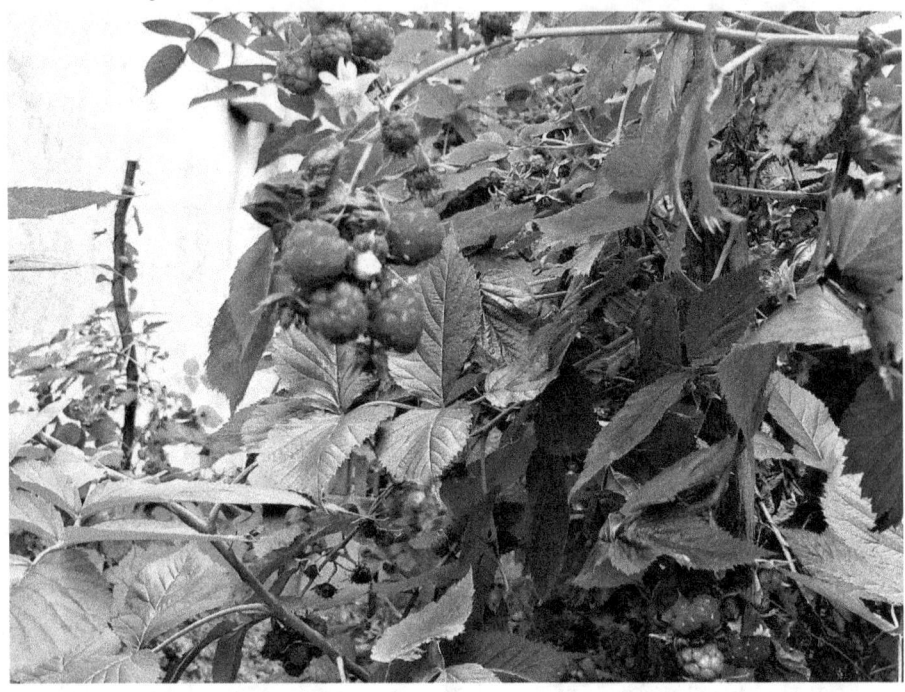

It is a perennial plant with green leaves and red edible fruits.

Red raspberries contain folate or vitamin B9. The synthetic version of folate is the folate acid. Folate has an important role in tissue and cell growth, it reduces the risk of stroke, it is good for colon health, supports neural health, supports normal fetal development, promotes sperm viability and it is great for heart problems.

Red raspberries protects the liver, they have antioxidant anti-inflammatory properties and they have the ability to destroy the stomach and colon cancer cells. The fruits contain vitamin C, E, K; fibers, biotin, pantothenic acid, omega 3 fats, folates, tannins and minerals like manganese, potassium, magnesium and copper.

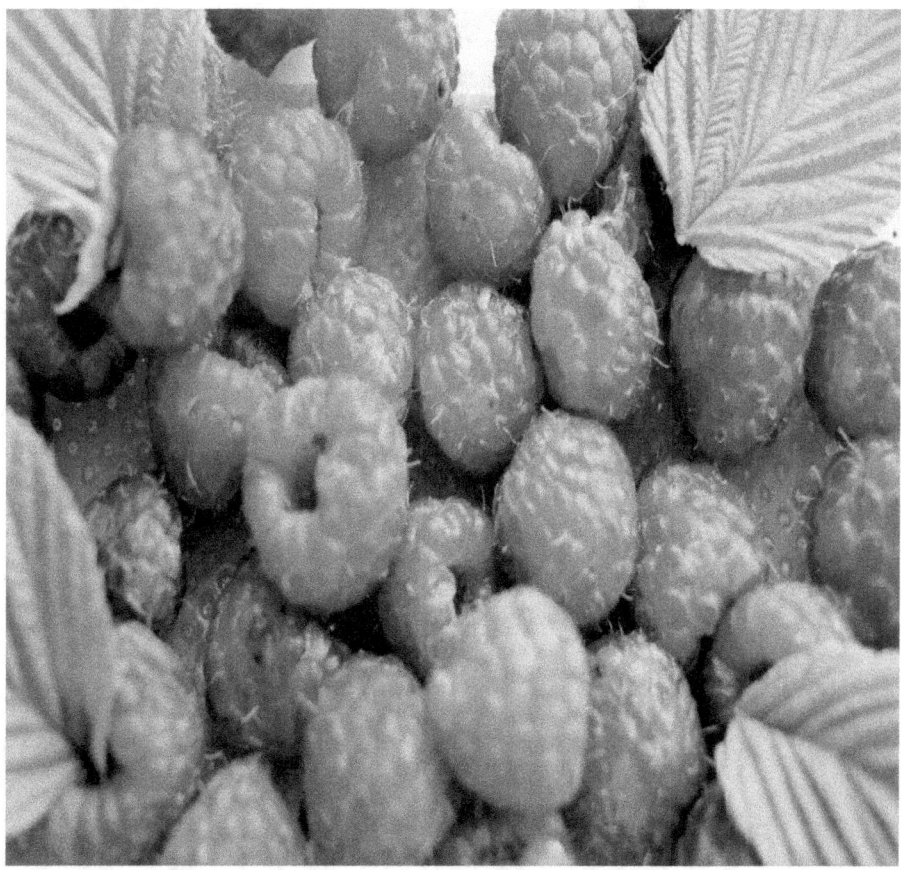

The raspberry leaves are used with success in diarrhea, mouthwashes (a gargle to treat tonsillitis and mouth inflammations because of their astringent action), it relieves the uterus muscles during labor, help menstrual cramps. The leaves are also used as an irrigation for burns, sores and varicose vein ulcers, morning sickness, in respiratory infections, in case of fever to promote sweating.

How to prepare the raspberry tea

Add 2 fresh, chopped raspberry leaves and 5 raspberries in a cup, pour boiling water and let steep for 2 minutes.

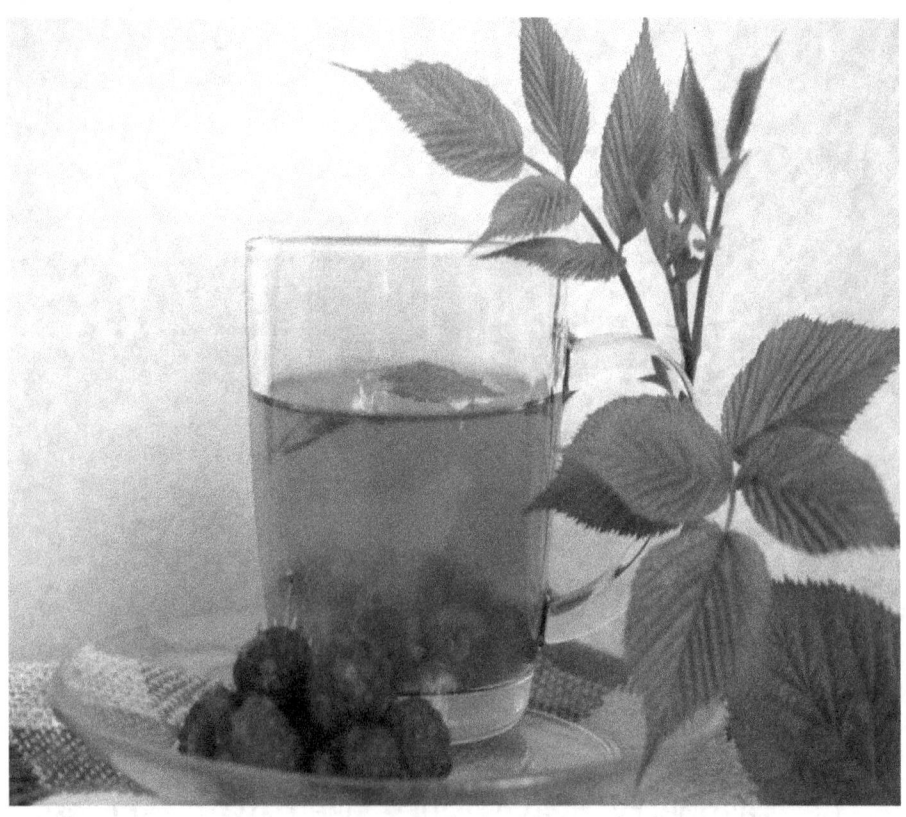

For a tea made with dried leaves and fruits, add 1 teaspoon of dried raspberry leaves and berries in a cup, pour boiling water and let steep for 2-3 minutes.

If your bird is suffering from vitamin C deficiency the raspberry tea is a very good choice for him/her.

This tea has beneficial properties if is consumed before and during egg laying periods, it also great to use if your bird is suffering from neural problems (when the bird is unable to hold itself properly on the perches, continuously shakes its head, etc...).

The males should consume this tea before mating periods, because the raspberry compounds promote sperm viability.

It is a very good tea which can be used in respiratory infections as well.

Blueberry (Vaccinium corymbosum)

Blueberry or Vaccinium corymbosum is a perennial plant of genus Vaccinium in the family Ericaceae. Blueberries are native to North America, but today this plant can be found all over the world. The blueberry shrubs have indigo almost black color fruits and green, ovate or lanceolate leaves and can grow from 10 cm (3.9 in) to 4 metres (13 ft) high.

The larger species of blueberries are known as highbush blueberries and the smaller species are known as lowbush blueberries. There are several species of blueberries: Bilberry or European blueberry (Vaccinium myrtillus), Evergreen blueberry (Vaccinium darrowii), Alaskan blueberry (Vaccinium alaskaense), New Jersey blueberry (Vaccinium caesariensis), Hillside blueberry (Vaccinium constablaei), Costa Rican blueberry (Vaccinium consanguineum), Shiny blueberry Vaccinium myrsinites, etc...

Blueberries contain proteins, carbohydrates, antioxidants, vitamin A, B1 (thiamine), B2 (riboflavin), B3 (niacin), B5 (pantothenic acid), B6, B9 (folate), C, E, K, minerals like phosphorus, manganese, iron, calcium, potassium, magnesium, sodium and zinc. They also contain phytochemicals as anthocyanins, polyphenols.

Avoid buying varieties of blueberry teas that contain black tea leaves and blueberry flavors, as they contain caffeine. Just make sure that you are purchasing the correct variety of this type of tea from the store.

How to prepare the blueberry tea
Add 8 chopped, fresh leaves and 8 fresh berries in a mug, pour boiling water and steep for 2 minutes.

When preparing tea with dried leaves and berries, add 1 teaspoon of dried berries and leaves in a cup, pour boiling water and let steep for 2-3 minutes.

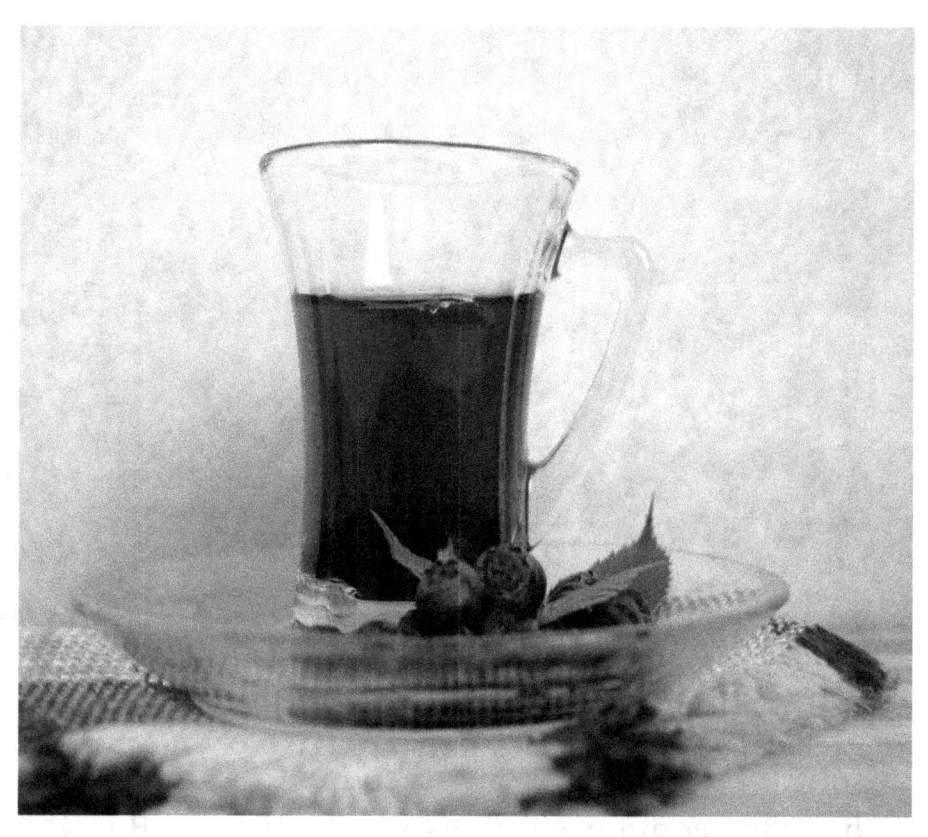

Rose hips

Rose hips are the fruits of a deciduous shrub called Rosa Canina, Dog Rose or Wild Rose. This plant is native to Europe, Africa and Asia and belong to the family Rosaceae. The stems are covered with sharp prickles, the pinnate leaves are green, the flowers are pale pink color, the red to orange colored fruits are called rose hips.

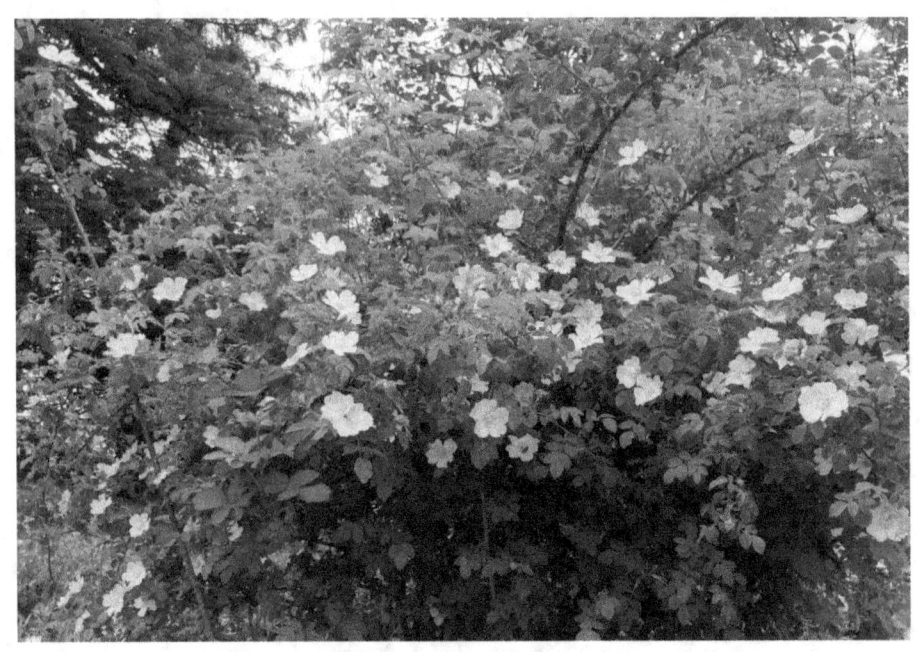

Blooming Wild Rose flowers

Rose hips have a very high content of vitamin C but they also contain vitamins like A, B1, B2, B3, K and minerals like iron, calcium, magnesium, manganese, selenium, zinc, potassium, sulphur, phosphorus, It also contains pectin, tannin, flavonoids, lycopene, lutein, beta-carotene and zeaxanthin. The rose hips extract helps reduce arthritis pain, it has diuretic action and helps with digestion, lower cholesterol, it is a great remedy against respiratory problems, manage diabetes, it is a good immune system booster, increase urination and help in building stronger bones, prevent cancer and keeps skin healthy.

Rose hips tea can be used especially during Winter, but it is also good to be offered as a refresher all year long. Vitamin C intake is always welcoming for your birds.

In cold season you can moisten your bird`s seeds with some cod liver oil, which contains a high level of fat, protein and vitamin D. It is a supplement that should be given occasionally to the birds by helping them especially during Winter. This recommendation is for those birds that are likely to be kept in outdoor aviaries.

How to prepare the rose hips tea

Add 1 teaspoon of dried rose hips in a cup, pour boiling water, steep for 3-4 minutes and strain.

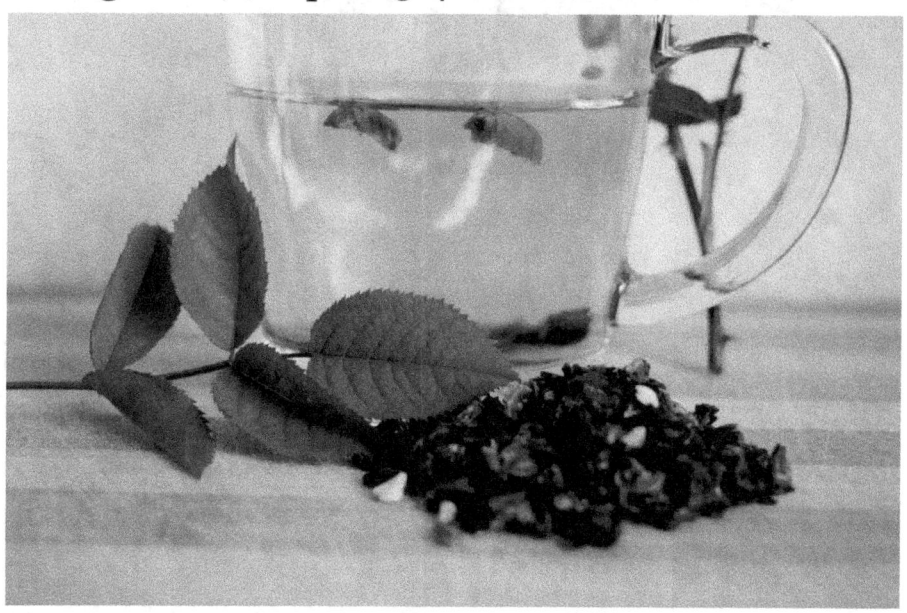

When preparing tea with fresh herb, add 8 fresh, chopped rose hips in a cup, pour boiling water, steep for 2-3 minutes and strain it well.

Blackcurrant (Ribes nigrum)

The blackcurrant is a woody shrub in the family Grossulariaceae. It has green leaves and very dark purple almost black, piquant berries.

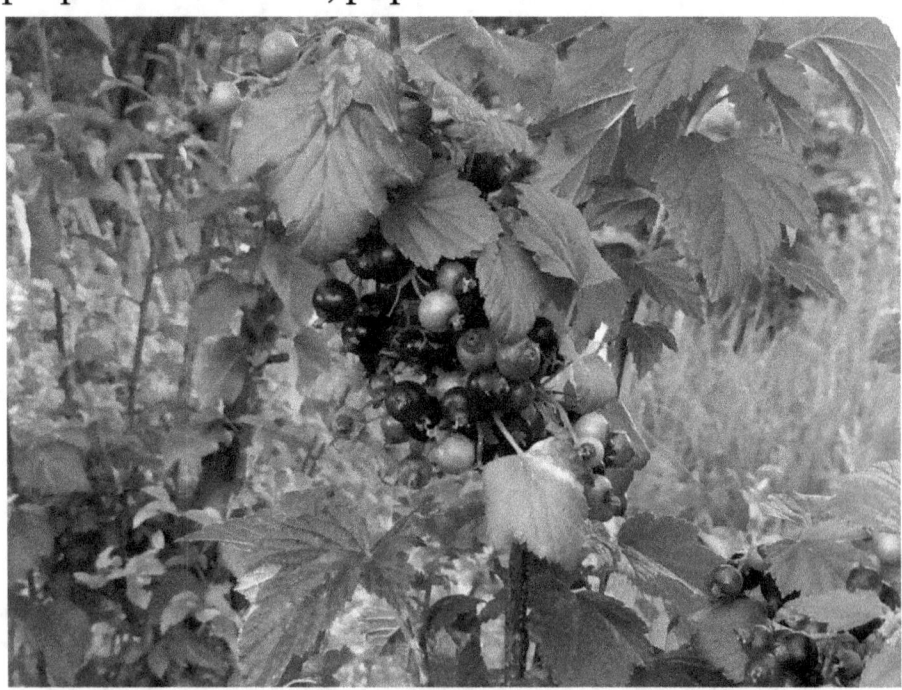

It is native to central and northern Europe and Asia. The berries contain high level of vitamin C, E, B1 (thiamine), B2 riboflavin, B3 niacin, B5 (pantothenic acid, B6, polyphenol phytochemicals (in fruits, seeds and leaves), pectins, acids, minerals like iron, manganese, calcium, magnesium, phosphorus, potassium, zinc, sodium. Blackcurrants have higher level of vitamin C than oranges.

Blackcurrant seed oil contain vitamin E, fatty acids like alpha linolenic acid, gamma linolenic acid.

Blackcurrant is an immune system booster, it has anti-inflammatory properties, treats infection, protects against influenza, anti-cancer benefits especially liver cancer, treats anaemia, microbial infections, it helps lower cardiovascular diseases.

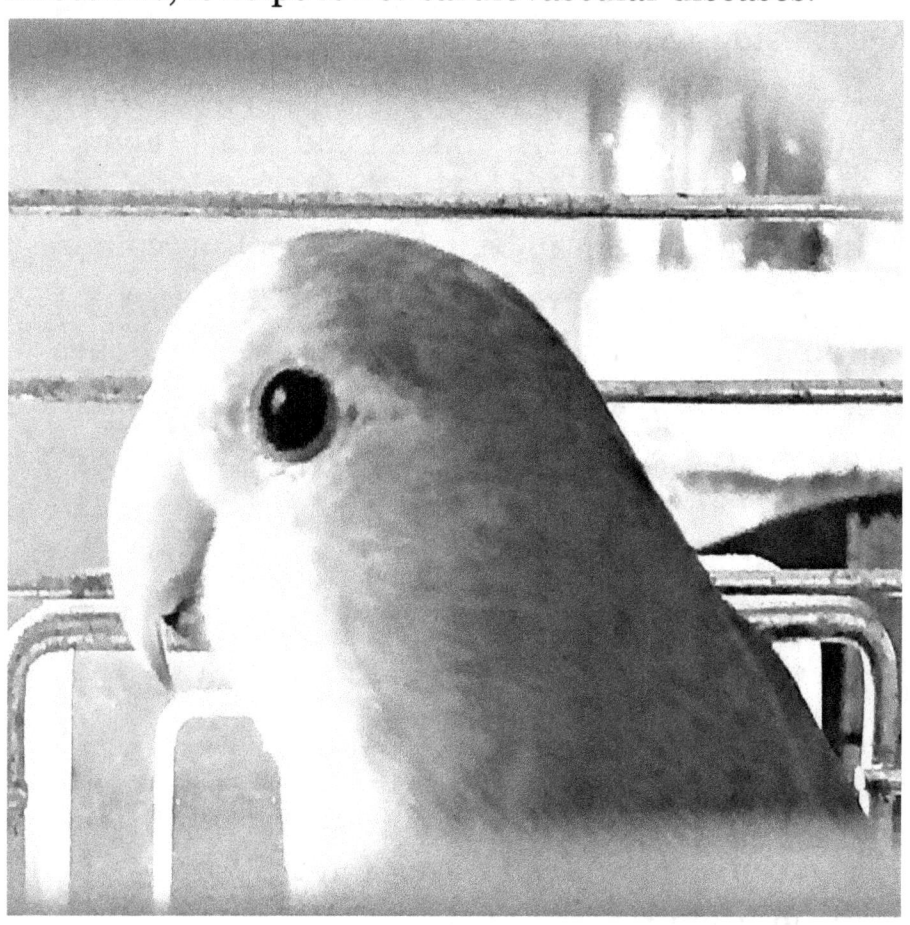

The skin of the blackcurrant fruit is rich in anthocyanins, compound that slow down the growth of the cancer cells.

The leaves have diuretic properties, improves the function of the kidneys and liver, and treats the kidney stones, improves mental health and stress level, it also has vermifuge properties.

The blackcurrant tea is beneficial for skin problems like eczemas and dermatitis because of its internal cleansing action.

If your bird is suffering from visual problems like blurry vision, then you should start giving this aromatic tea to your bird.

Blackcurrant tea can be used externally as compresses for poorly healing wounds and insect bites.

Too much blackcurrant tea can cause diarrhea and gastrointestinal problems, therefore you should offer your bird this tea only 2 times per day for 2-3 days.

Avoid buying varieties of blackcurrant teas that contain black tea leaves and black currant flavors, as they contain caffeine. Just make sure that you are purchasing the correct variety of this type of tea from the store.

How to prepare the blackcurrant tea
You can use the fresh leaves and the fruits as well for the infusion.

Add 1 chopped, green leaf and 8-10 berries in a cup, pour boiling water and steep for 5 minutes.

When you prepare the tea from dried leaves and berries, use 1 teaspoon of dried leaves and berries for a cup of boiling water and let steep for 3 minutes.

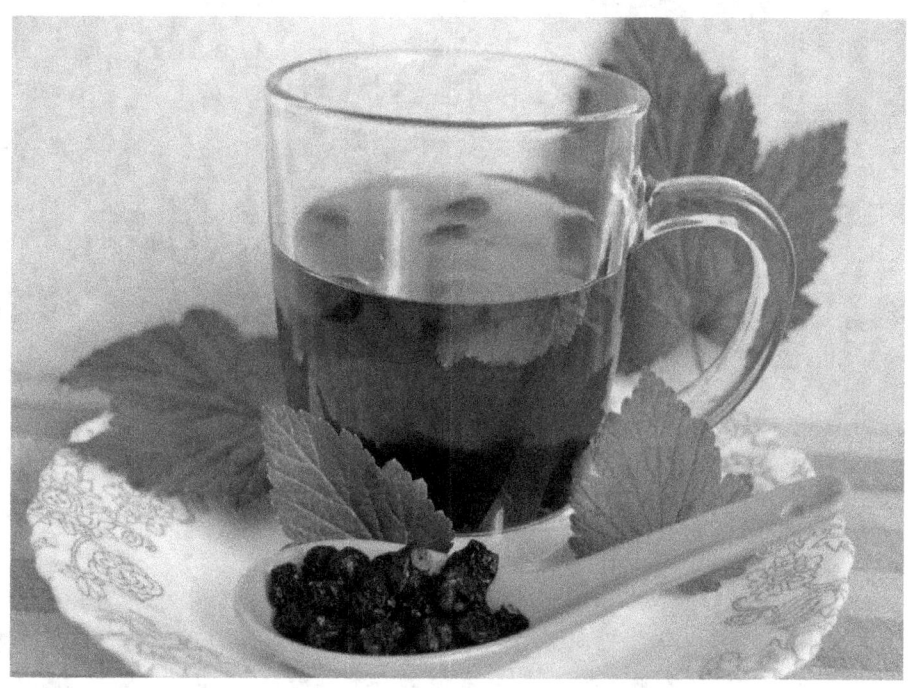

Ribwort plantain (Plantago lanceolata)

Plantago lanceolata or Ribwort plantain is a perennial flowering plant in the family Plantaginaceae. It is also called ribgrass and is native to Europe and Asia, although it can be found almost all over the world. This plant has dark green lanceolate leaves with 3-5 strong, parallel veins and flowering stalks, which are arranged in a dense rosette. The flower head is ovoid and sits on top of a wiry flower stalk.

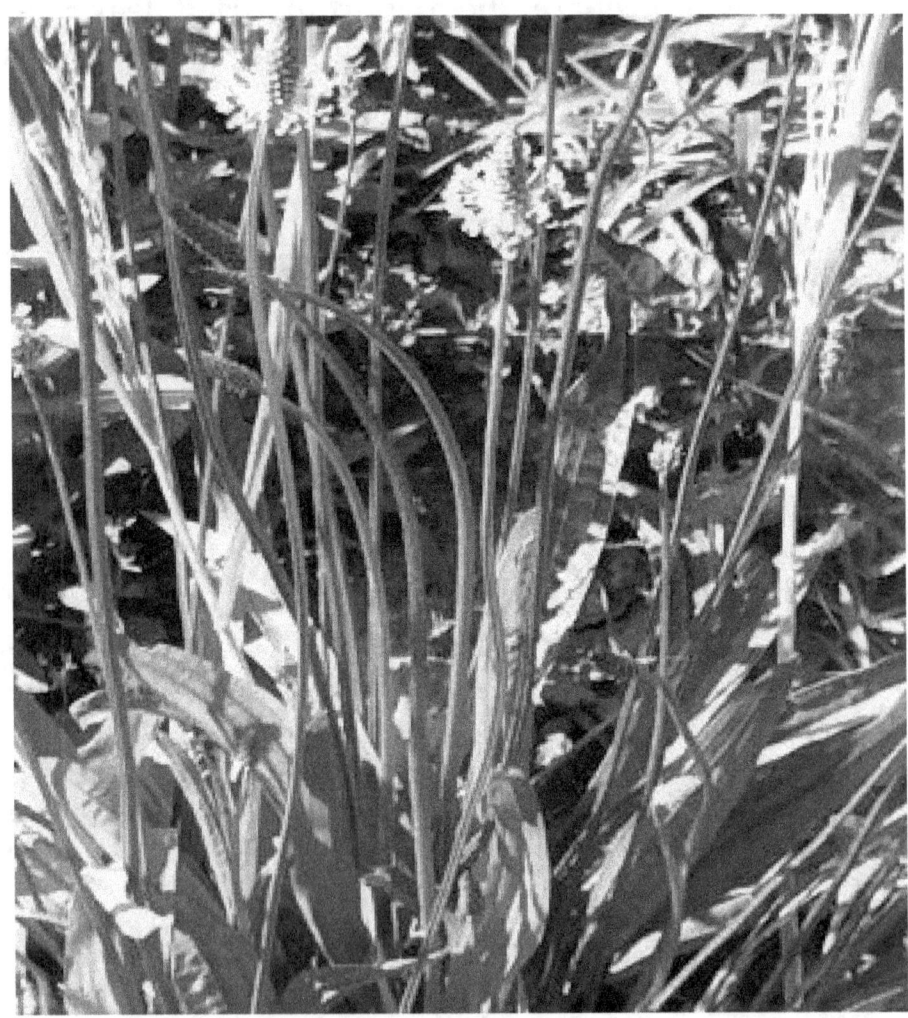

There are two different types of plantain: Ribwort or Narrow-leaf (Plantago lanceolata) and Broadleaf (Plantago major). These plants have the same chemical composition and both types are great natural remedies.

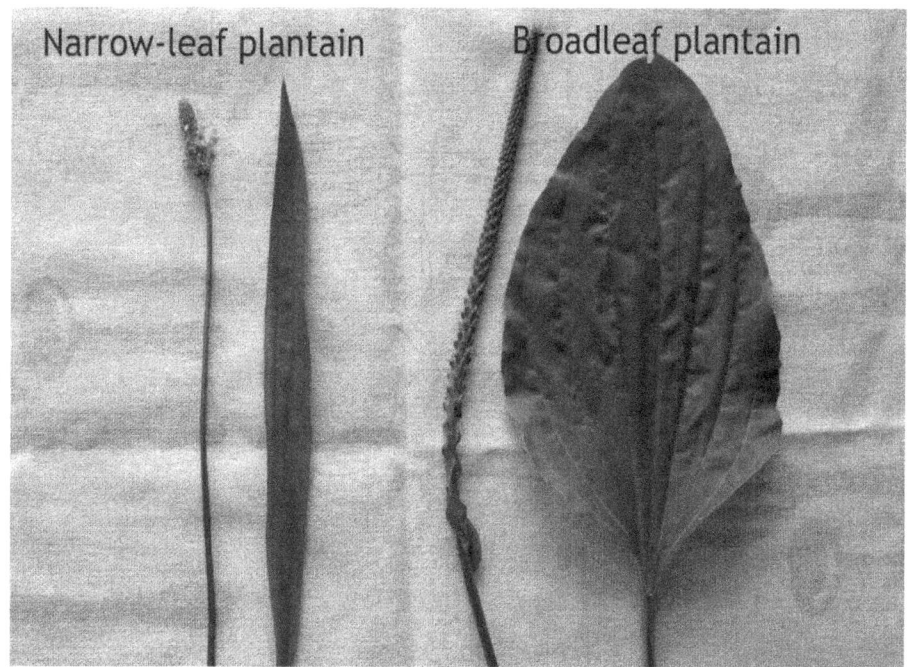

Narrow-leaf plantain   Broadleaf plantain

The fresh, young leaves are edible and can be used raw in salads or it also can be cooked in the same manner as spinach.

Ribwort plantain contains vitamin A, C, K, iron, calcium, phenolic acids, allantoin, coumarins, flavonoids, ursolic acids, glycosides and volatile oils. It also has anti-inflammatory, antioxidant, astringent, wound healing, analgesic, anti-ulcerogenic and immune system booster properties.

The tea made from Plantain leaves treat gout, which helps excreting the increased uric acid from the kidneys. Plantain tea also treats diarrhoea and as a result of the high vitamin and mineral content of this plant, it simultaneously reestablishes the nutrients lost as a result of diarrhoea.

The plantain seeds have laxative properties, so you can use them to treat constipation.

This herb can be used internally as teas or externally for treatment of the skin like insect bites and infections, for dry cough, wound healing, gum and loosen tooth.

The Ribwort tea is a very efficient remedy against respiratory tract infections, urinary tract infections and painful ulcers in human.

When using externally, the fresh leaves should be applied as compresses on the affected areas of the skin.

For skin burn, crush 1-2 fresh leaves and apply them on the affected area. Cover with an adhesive gauze bandage. This plant will help relieve the pain and will help with the regeneration of the new skin cells.

The fresh, crushed leaves can heal and relieve the pain of the swollen lymph node. It also helps stop bleeding.

For itching skin and feather picking problems, just spray your bird with lukewarm plantain tea every morning, until the bird is healed.

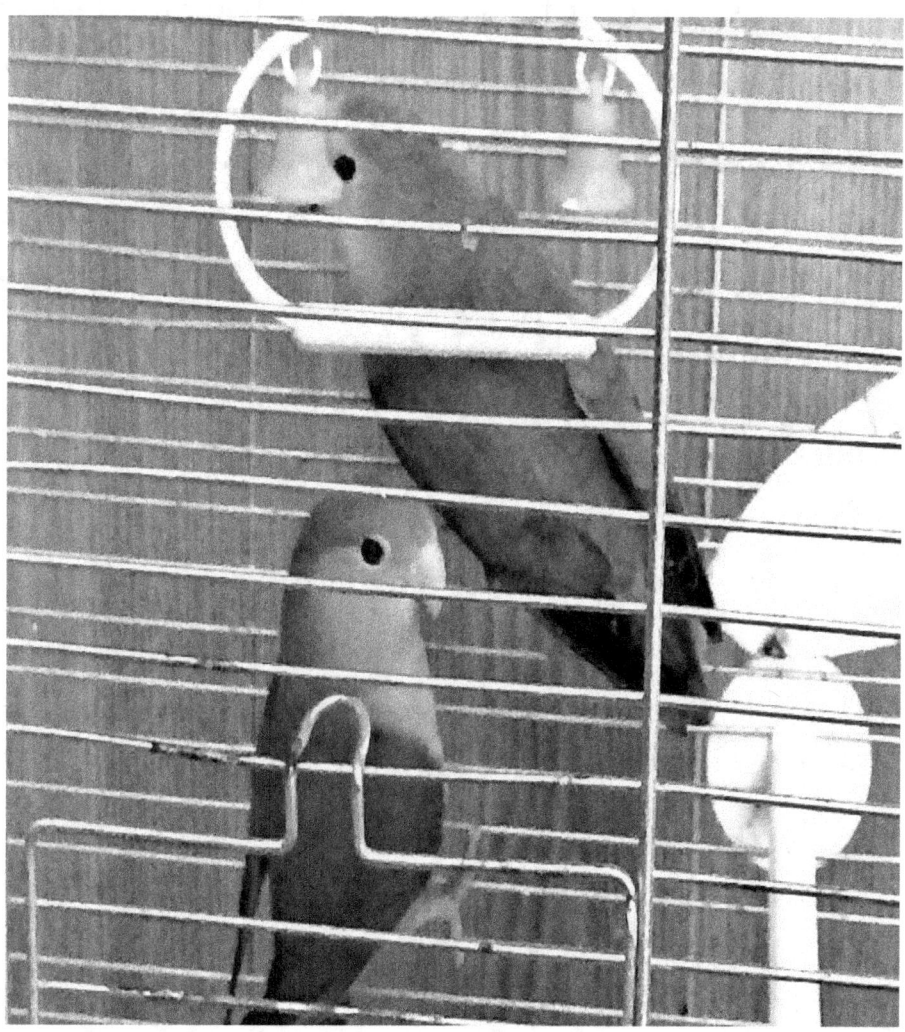

The freshly chewed plantain works on gums and teeth and also on ripped toenail in humans.

If your bird`s nails are injured or ripped off, just try the following application:

Get a fresh plantain leaf and put it in a mug. Pour boiling water over the leaf. Let it sit two minutes until soft and bright green, then run the leaf under cool water until it is cool. Wrap the toe with the leaf and bandage it. You will need to change the leaf much more often so it does not dry out. It has very good anti inflammatory properties and also a perfect pain relief.

The ribwort plantain oil can be used with success in the treatment of dry skin, chicken pox or avian pox, burns, dermatitis, bee stings, eczema, snake bites, etc...

How to prepare the Ribwort plantain oil

Fill a jar with dried or fresh Ribwort plantain leaves (fresh leaves are better), pour olive oil on them, use a spoon to gently stir the plants and seal the jar.

Allow the leaves and oil to steep for 2-3 weeks. Gently shake the jar every few days to encourage the plants to release their beneficial compounds. After 2-3 weeks, strain the oil through a cheesecloth. Try to wring the cheesecloth well and tight to make sure that you get every drop of this wonderful oil. Store the plantain oil in a dark-colored glass bottle with a tight-fitting cap.

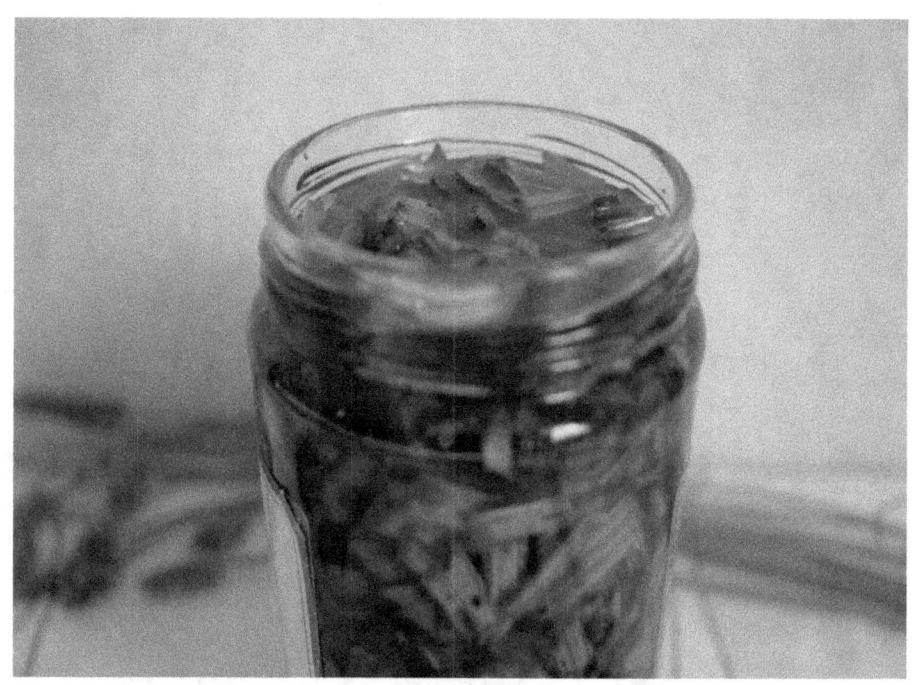

If your bird is suffering from various skin problems, then you can definitely use this wonderful oil. It can be used to treat swellings and lesions on the bird`s legs and feet. Apply the oil on the affected area 2-3 times per day until the wound is healed.

How to prepare the Plantain tea

Add 2-3 chopped, fresh Plantain leaves in a cup, pour boiling water and let steep for 30 seconds or 1 minute.

When preparing the tea with dried herbs, add 1 teaspoon of dried herbs in a cup, pour boiling water and let steep for 1-2 minutes.

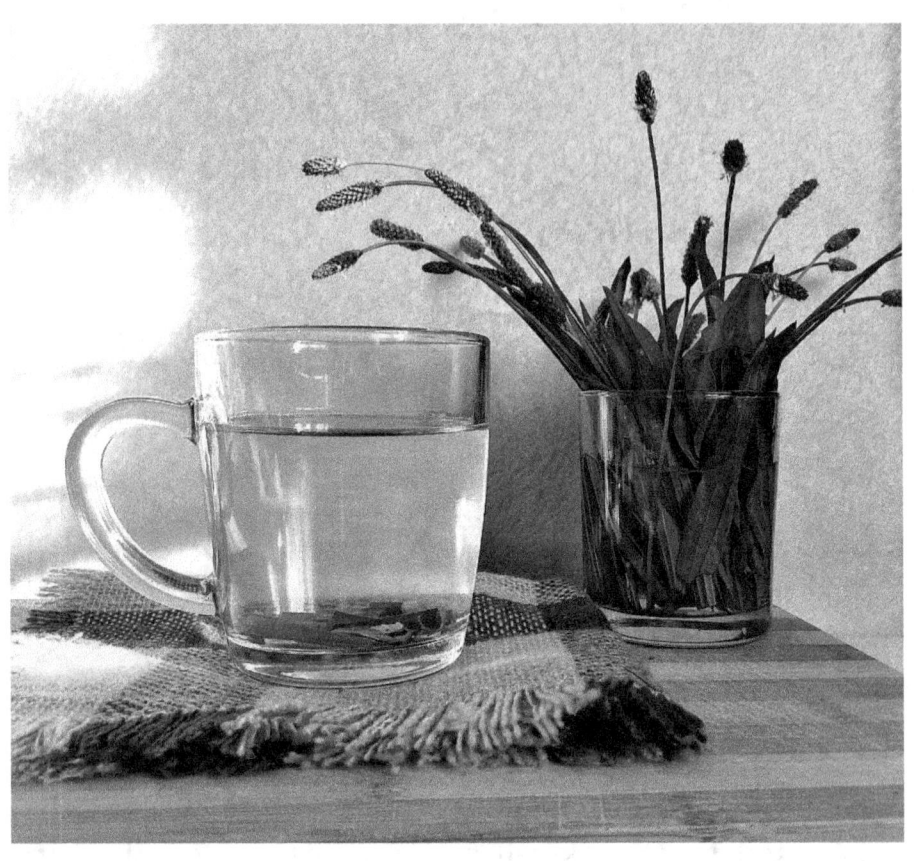

Constipation

If your bird is suffering from constipation, the cloacal orifice free opening is needed by administering few drops of castor oil through the bird's beak, for two-three days. The bird will need a warm place and for the next few days the diet will contain honey, green plants, plantain seeds, fruits and chamomile tea. If the chamomile tea doesn't work, replace it with plantain tea made from seeds: add 1 teaspoon of fresh or dried seeds in a cup, pour boiling water and let steep for 2-3 minutes. This tea can be added in the bird's drinking bowls 3 times per day for a week.

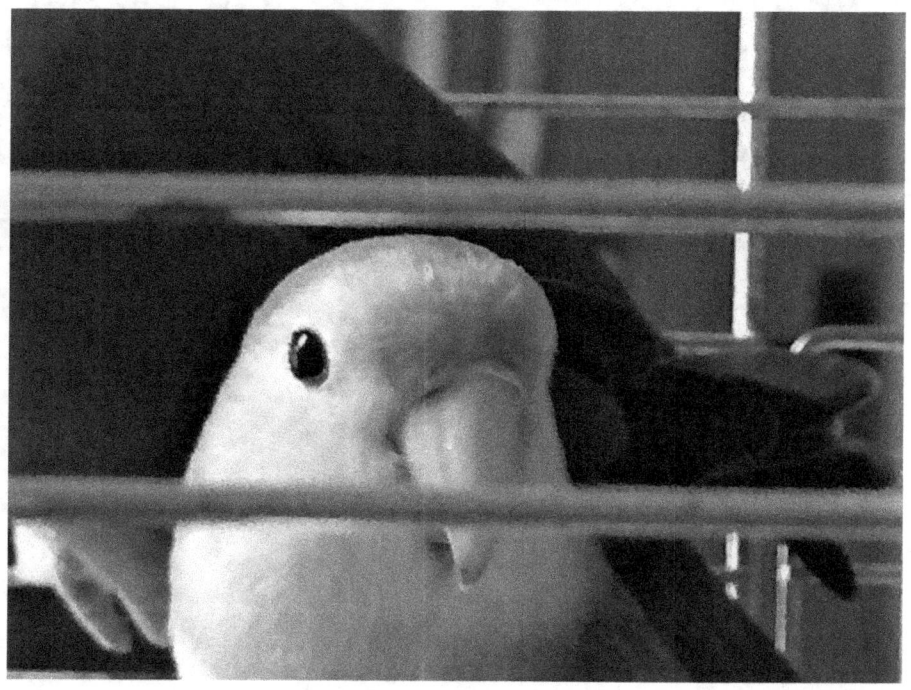

Shepherd's purse (Capsella bursa - pastoris)

Shepherd's purse or Capsella bursa - pastoris is an annual flowering plant in the family Brassicaceae. It is native to Europe and Asia, but today it is considered a common weed all over the world. This plant has small, white flowers and purse like green fruits that are triangular shaped and flat. The lobed leaves can be found at the base of the plant.

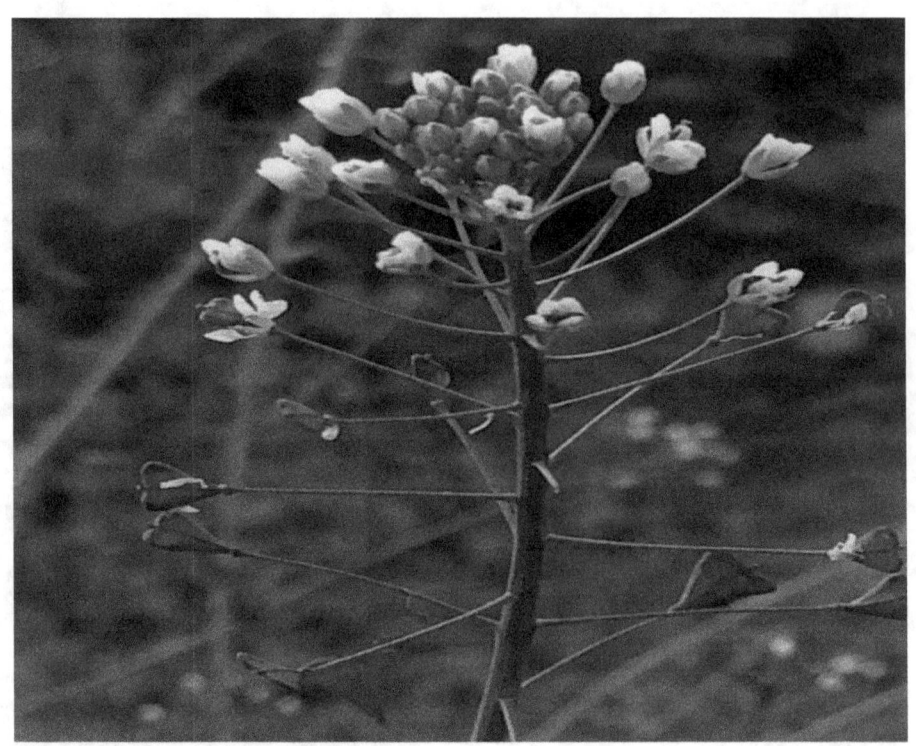

Shepherd's purse contains various amines as histamine, tyramine, acetylcholine, choline; flavonoids; glycosides; essential oils, sinigrin, carotenoids, vitamins A, B, C and K and minerals as potassium, manganese, copper, iron, calcium, phosphorus,

It has anti-inflammatory properties and it relieves the pain of rheumatism, it is also good in treatment of muscle atrophy.

The Shepherd's purse is recommended for internal and external bleeding. Internally it can be used after egg laying period when there is blood present in the urine or in the droppings.

This plant is used externally to heal minor wounds and cuts and it is also good for hemorrhoids and varicose veins. The tea made from this herb has beneficial effects in treatments of sore throat, urinary tract infection, earache, chronic diarrhea, it also improves eyesight and vision.

To stop nasal bleeding just insert into the nostrils a cotton swab dipped in the Shepherd's purse infusion.

If your bird is suffering from muscle atrophy you should prepare the following infusion for internal and external use (massage the affected areas with this infusion):

How to prepare the Shepherd's purse tea
Add 1 teaspoon of fresh, chopped shepherd`s purse in a cup, pour boiling water and steep for 1 minutes.

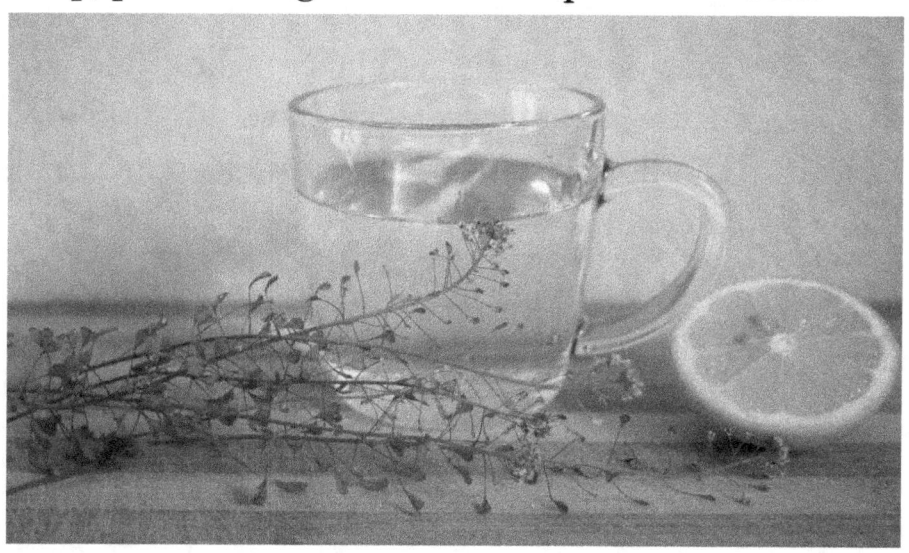

When preparing the tea with dried herbs, add 1 teaspoon of dried plant in a cup, pour boiling water and steep for 2 minutes.

Disclaimer

The author accepts no responsibility for any loss or injury, as a result for the use or misuse of the information in this book. Before you decide to use any of the remedies presented in this book, make sure to consult with your qualified avian vet or with a qualified physician. Mixing the plants together or if your bird is taking other medication, you want to be cautious!

Before considering any guidance from this book, please ensure your bird do not have any underlying health conditions which may interfere with the suggested healing methods.

I hope this book will help you keep your birds happy and healthy and it is been a pleasure for me to write it down for you.

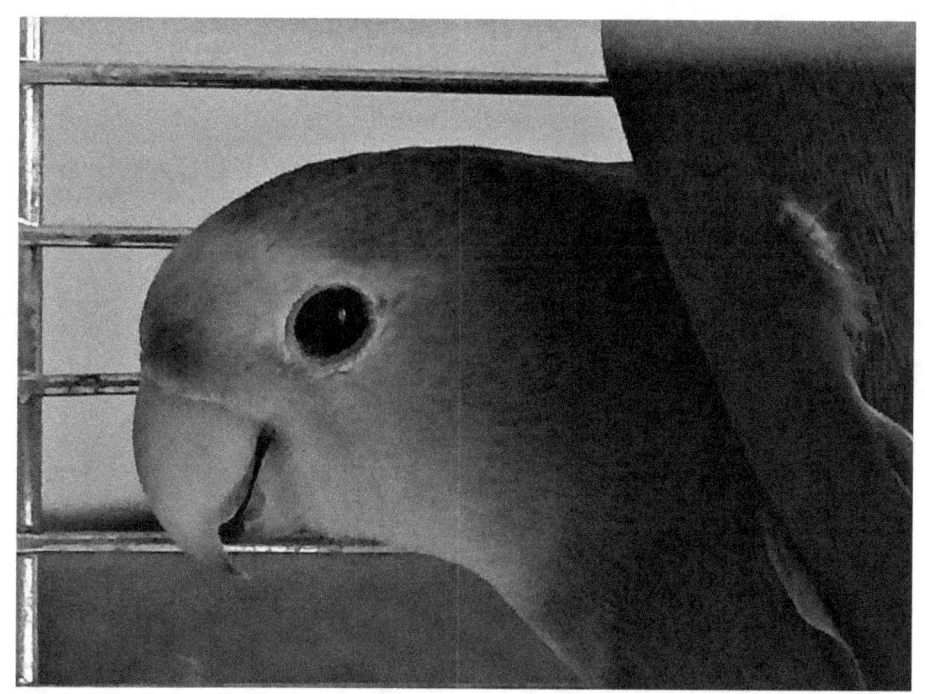

Please check the following page where you can find my other writings:

More from the author

You can find all these books on Amazon.com.

Brought to you by Erika Busecan